"I was so encouraged by what was said."
Sheila Walsh, CBN "700 Club"

"See how you can take charge of your health care."
Gayle King, NBC "Cover to Cover"

*Every Parent's Nightmare*, by Annette and Dan Tomal, is an extremely vital book for everyone to read. It describes the "limitless responsibility" that all parents should feel for their offspring no matter what the disability. If all parents in the world showed the love and active concern of the Tomals for the well-being of their child, it would mark a new milennium."
Alfred Swanson, M.D.,
Director of Orthopaedic Surgery
Residency Training Program
Grand Rapids Hospitals

"To survive, we must do our homework—the Tomals certainly did theirs, and in recording it have given us a map, a spirit, and an attitude. In my skiing career such moments of pain and crisis have also been a vehicle of awakening."
Susy Chaffee,
Olympic Ski Team Captain,
World Free-Style Champion

"Jonathan Tomal's story is both an inspiration to anyone who has ever faced adversity and a dark reminder that tragedy can overcome the lives of any family. But the perseverance of the Tomal family as told in this book will not be forgotten and has created a movement to ensure that other families do not need to follow in their footsteps, frantically searching for a cure."
U.S. Representative Tim Roemer (D) Indiana

"Here are two marvelous books for the price of one! The story is next to impossible to put down. The lessons learned by the Tomals in finding the right medical assistance become a great help to all of us."
David and Karen Mains, The Chapel of the Air

"The Tomals' story clearly demonstrates what happens when medical consumers, not fully informed by their doctors about choices and treatments, take matters into their own hands. When their son was first diagnosed with an inoperable brain tumor, local doctors, as well as a major medical center, told them to enjoy what time was left. The Tomals refused to accept this verdict and set about finding the one neurosurgeon who saved their child. Their inspirational story is proof positive that medicine is far more of an art than a science. And their persistence in seeking other opinions should be a lesson to us all."

Charles B. Inlander, President, People's Medical Society

"Be inspired and informed . . ."
Myrna Blyth, *Ladies' Home Journal.*

"Within any organization or family there is always some level of dysfunctional behavior and structure. The Tomals have both lived and told a story naming some of the myths and pathology within the medical community. Their story is empowering to us and a helpful self-study for the profession."

Rick Chaffee, U.S. Olympic Ski Team 1968, 1972

". . . puts a personal face on the high technology that saves lives every day."
Phyllis Piano, Manager,
Communication and Community Relations
GE Medical Systems

"*Every Parent's Nightmare* is for everyone who has ever shared the pain of an innocent child, or placed exaggerated faith in the omniscience of doctors. Reading this deeply touching and enlightening book is an epiphany."
Jeff Lyon, *Chicago Tribune Sunday Magazine.
Author, *Playing God in the Nursery*

# Every Parent's Nightmare

## A Young Family's Triumph Over Their Son's Critical Illness

## Daniel R. & Annette Tomal
### Foreword by Ben Carson, M.D.

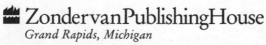 Zondervan Publishing House
*Grand Rapids, Michigan*

*A Division of* HarperCollins*Publishers*

Requests for information should be addressed to:
Zondervan Publishing House
Grand Rapids, Michigan 49530

The publisher and authors are not medical doctors and are therefore not licensed to provide medical advice. All sources in this book (associations, hospitals, physicians, government agencies, clinics, and the like) are not intended to be an endorsement or a recommendation. Readers are to use their own judgment, along with their physicians, for their medical care. No liability is assumed with respect to the use of the information herein.

Library of Congress Cataloging-in-Publication Data

Tomal, Daniel R.
    Every parent's nightmare : a young family's fight to save their child's life / Daniel R. and Annette Tomal.
      p.  cm.
    Includes biographical references.
    ISBN 0-310-59821-4 (paper)
    1. Tomal, Jonathan, 1980—Health. 2. Tumors in children—
Patients—Ohio—Biography. 3. Brain—Tumors—Patients—Ohio—
Biography. 4. Physicians. 5. Consumer education. I. Tomal,
Annette. II. Title.
RC281.C4T63  1993
362.1'10973—dc20                               93–42785
                                                              CIP

*Edited by Mary McCormick*
*Cover designed by The Aslan Group*
*Cover illustration by Patrick Kelley*

*Printed in the United States of America*

93  94  95  96  97  98  99 / DH / 10  9  8  7  6  5  4  3  2  1

*To the parents and medical practitioners
who truly understand.
God bless you.*

# Contents

# Appendices

# Foreword

When one of your young children is diagnosed with a very serious or even terminal disease process, you feel as though someone has "pulled the rug out" from beneath you. Suddenly, your title, possessions, and almost everything else lose their significance for you, and you are willing to give anything or do anything to save your child. *Every Parent's Nightmare* vividly captures this feeling of despair as well as the subsequent emotional and rational thought processes that allowed the Tomal family to survive an often irrational and self-serving medical system and to eventually claim triumph by doing their best and letting God do the rest.

In my own practice, I have frequently encountered distraught parents whose sick child has been written off by local medical authorities. Like the Tomals, these families have persevered and resisted the urge to give up, and in many of the cases, solutions were found. This book is very important because after establishing a connection with the needy reader, it supplies extremely practical solutions for overcoming the many roadblocks that lie between the medically needy and the best medical facilities and expertise in the world.

I would be thrilled if every medical student in the United States were required to read this book, because it is important for physicians to understand the distress that they themselves frequently cause, perhaps unintentionally, by adopting self-serving attitudes and yielding to professional peer pressure. It requires a supremely confident and compassionate medical specialist to refer a difficult problem to someone else in his/her own specialty, since this requires an admission or at least the consideration of possible personal inadequacy to solve the problem. Obviously, this is the wrong way to view the situation inasmuch as not everyone will have the same amount of experience, facilities, or back-up personnel to apply to every problem. I hope and believe that more of us in the medical profession now understand that God has put us here to help bring about healing of the body, mind, and spirit rather than to pursue self-aggrandizement.

The practical information contained in this book, including names, addresses, and telephone numbers is difficult to find and can save the reader many frustrating hours of intense labor. The approach to finding the right doctor is very well-balanced and fair. It should also be emphasized that one of the most valuable resources that you can find to determine the appropriateness of your choice of medical specialists and facilities is other patients and families who have utilized them. If you are in doubt, do not hesitate to ask for references. If this offends the physician, that should raise a red flag.

Finally, I am rejoicing along with many others because the Tomal family found Dr. Fred Epstein, who is not only an outstanding pediatric neurosurgeon but a very fine human being who personally took the time to encourage me early in my career. I hope that all the readers of this book will find the encouragement, inspiration, and faith needed to tackle not only medical problems but all the problems of life.

— Benjamin Carson, M.D.
Director of Pediatric Neurosurgery:
Johns Hopkins Hospital

# *Acknowledgments*

Many people have contributed directly or indirectly to bringing our story to print.

We first thank God for providing us with the strength and courage to resolve Jonathan's medical problem. We thank our parents, family, friends, and church family for supporting us during that difficult time. We especially recognize Dr. Fred Epstein and the New York University Medical Center, and we particularly acknowledge the courage of our son Jonathan throughout his painful hospitalization and recovery.

We thank Ellie Grossman for her encouragement and her article about our story in *Ladies' Home Journal*. We thank Harry Smith of CBS "This Morning," Gayle King and Niles Jaeger of NBC "Cover to Cover," Pat Robertson, Sheila Walsh, and David Gyertson of CBN "700 Club," General Electric Medical Systems, Congressmen Tim Roemer and Henry Waxman, John St. Croix, Estelle Tomal, Gladys Crowl, George Sewitt, and so many other people who provided us with the inspiration to continue writing. We give our very special thanks to Dr. Ben Carson for his genuine help and support in writing the foreword to this book.

We are most indebted to Zondervan Publishing House and to Lyn Cryderman, who believed in this story and took it to print. Finally, we give our heartfelt appreciation to so many parents across the country who have called to share their stories about their own children's suffering from brain tumors. These parents truly understand the pain, suffering, and frustrations of trying to save our children in the midst of the ineffective medical referral system in our country. We thank those parents who kept urging us to continue "spreading the word" even as their own children were dying. We respect them and applaud them for their courage and commitment.

# Part One
## Jonathan's Story

# Introduction

This book is about our son, who was diagnosed with a brain tumor when he was not quite four years old—initially given a prognosis of just months to live. His doctor told us that there was nothing that could be done to help our son. We were, however, determined to fight the medical referral system and were able to finally find a doctor who did help our son, who is now a perfectly normal twelve-year-old with no tumor whatsoever left.

Because we don't feel that anyone should have to go through what we did to find the proper medical treatment, we have written this book—to provide inspiration as well as direction. The first part of this book is "Jonathan's Story," detailing our experiences trying to find the doctor who saved Jonathan's life. The second part will give you guidance and direction as you try to find the "right" doctor for whatever medical problem you have.

For ease of reading, we have written "Jonathan's Story" in the third person. Every word, every emotion, is ours, however. We hope that the story will inspire you to take charge of your own medical problem and that Part Two will show you how to do so. God's charge to us to treat our body as a temple means that we *must take charge* of our medical treatment.

# 1

# The Shocking Diagnosis

*A person flipping through the pages* of the Tomals' photo album would find photographs remarkably similar to photographs in thousands of other photo albums around the country. The same milestones would be recorded . . . the same events, just with different faces . . . a baby's first step . . . a family vacation . . . a visit from Santa Claus . . . a day at the beach . . . everyday, ordinary events in the lives of millions of people throughout the country.

A person could follow the history of the Tomal family by going through their photo albums: the wedding of Dan and Annette in 1973 in the small town of Three Oaks, Michigan; their graduation from Ball State University in 1974; their first apartment and their first jobs, as high school teachers in Joliet, Illinois; building a new house a couple of years later; moving to Ohio for Dan to pursue his Ph.D.; the birth of Jonathan in 1980; many, many pictures of his infancy and toddlerhood; the birth of Stephanie in 1984. The photo albums show the typical flow of many middle-class lives— from college to marriage to careers to children.

September 1983 shows Jonathan ready for his first day of nursery school—three and one-half years old, blond hair cut in a "Dutch bowl" style, big grin on his face, dressed in a red-and-blue striped shirt and red shorts, standing on the porch of a typical two-story frame-and-brick middle-class home. A favorite after-school activity was dressing up in a

17

football uniform and playing with the other neighbor boys, also in uniform. October 1984 shows Jonathan frolicking in the leaves in his backyard with his baby sister, Stephanie. That year for Halloween, Jonathan dressed up as the popular TV cartoon character, "He-Man." A picture shows Jonathan "helping" his dad install carpet in the dining room. Winter came early that year. A November picture shows a bundled-up Jonathan with several neighbor friends all grinning and throwing snowballs at the camera.

The next group of pictures shows a traditional Thanksgiving family get-together, with grandparents, aunts and uncles, and all the cousins—lots of laughter and smiles and hugs. The next page relates the annual Christmas preparation: Jonathan standing by the Christmas tree that he and his friends had just helped decorate; Jonathan in the kitchen with a neighbor girl helping make Christmas cookies; the annual Christmas-card picture—Jonathan with his mouth wide open as usual in a huge smile, blond hair shining, hazel eyes sparkling, his arms around dark-haired baby Stephanie.

A person might remark on the seemingly idyllic middle-class life the Tomals led. Both Dan and Annette were satisfied and fulfilled in their jobs. Dan had been a management consultant with Marathon Oil Company since finishing his Ph.D. before Jonathan's birth; Annette was a part-time instructor at Davis Business College. Dan and Annette had many friends and acquaintances in their small university town and were active church members. Dan frequently conducted Bible studies, helping apply Scripture to common, everyday problems in life; Annette regularly attended Bible studies and the Women's Circle group. She and the children were in a weekly play group with other young mothers. Jonathan had many friends in the neighborhood and regularly exchanged play dates with his nursery school friends. Dan would often remark, "I thank God that we have two such wonderful children" and would refer to Jonathan as "God's little angel." Yes, life was satisfying, fulfilling, and serene for the Tomals.

After November 1984 a person studying the Tomals' photo album would find many pictures startlingly different from those of other families. Pictures of Jonathan in the hospital . . . Jonathan celebrating his fourth birthday in the hospital . . . What happened in December had come as a complete shock to the family. One week after Thanksgiving, in the midst of the joyous Christmas preparations, Jonathan was diagnosed with a brain tumor. In only *one* day their world turned upside down and would never again be the same. The events leading to that fateful day, Tuesday, December 4, 1984, actually had begun just four days earlier.

Friday, November 30, began as had virtually every other Friday since August. Friday was a "fun day" for Annette and the kids—no work for Annette, who worked just two days a week, Mondays and Wednesdays, at the junior college. Annette found the balance between work and home extremely fulfilling. Her schedule also allowed her to be an active participant in the cooperative nursery school that Jonathan attended two mornings a week, Tuesdays and Thursdays. She was able to carpool with two other moms and also to work as a parent aide one morning a month.

The highlight of Fridays for Annette and the children was their weekly play group at different houses. When Jonathan was nine months old, a neighbor had asked Jonathan and Annette to join a play group she was forming. The children soon got into the routine of looking forward to Fridays to get together with their little friends, and the moms also soon began looking forward to the opportunity to relax over coffee and to chat about young-parent concerns. Remarkably, four of the five moms had had their second babies within four weeks of each other. The moms soon began joking that they looked forward to play group more than their kids did. An extremely close bond had been formed within the group of young mothers and their children.

That Friday passed uneventfully. As Annette prepared dinner, Jonathan was busy in the adjoining family room playing with his Matchbox cars; he loved lining them up or rolling them down the ramps of his Fisher-Price garage. He was such an organized little boy that he would get upset if someone rearranged his toys. He was unusually considerate of other people's feelings and had been saying "I'm sorry" and "Thank you" for over a year. He needed a warming-up period around new people but then would become quite friendly and would readily share his toys. Stephanie was sitting on the floor near Jonathan, picking up her toys and mouthing them. Jonathan adored Stephanie and was very concerned about her needs. He would regularly come to Annette and tell her, "Mommy, Stephanie's crying" or "Mommy, I think Stephanie's hungry."

As Annette was getting the dishes out of the cupboard to set the table, Jonathan said, "Mommy, my head hurts." Annette looked over at him, but he was so intent on his cars that she didn't even respond to his comment or mention it to Dan when he came home later that evening.

Saturday was fairly routine, with Dan and Annette doing their errands in the house and around town. As Dan and Annette relaxed in the family room that evening, Jonathan said, "Mommy, my head hurts." When Annette looked up at him, Jonathan was again intent on his cars, so again Annette didn't respond to his statement. Annette did comment to Dan, however, "You know, Dan, he said the same thing yesterday." Dan replied with frustration, "Oh, don't worry about it; everyone gets headaches." To himself, he thought,

*. . . So what? . . . Why is she trying to make something out of nothing?* Annette thought no more about it that evening.

Sunday started out somewhat hectic as usual . . . wanting to sleep in late . . . the mad rush to get everyone dressed in Sunday best, fed, and out the door in time for church. That afternoon, they took the children sledding. The town boasted only one sledding hill, made from the leftover dirt from the expressway built on the outskirts of town several years before. The hill was crowded with people but was still lots of fun for the kids.

That night at 3:00 A.M. Annette was awakened by loud crying. Always a light sleeper since Jonathan's birth, she jumped out of bed and rushed into his room. He was sitting up in bed, crying—"Mommy, my head hurts," to which Annette responded, "Okay, honey, just lie back down, and I'll get you some medicine." Annette gave him a chewable children's acetaminophen and laid him back down. Within a couple of minutes of stroking his back, Jonathan was asleep. Annette returned to bed and immediately fell back asleep, giving no more thought or concern to Jonathan. Dan hadn't even awakened.

The next day, Monday, was a workday for Annette, so she delivered Jonathan and Stephanie to their next-door neighbor, Debbie, who had been baby-sitting Jonathan since he was about two years old. The three headaches over the weekend had caused such little concern to Annette that she did not even mention them to Debbie.

The next morning, Tuesday, was nursery-school day for Jonathan. He woke up cheerfully, got dressed, and ate his favorite breakfast of Cheerios. Suddenly, he said "I don't feel good. My head hurts." Annette had him lie down on the couch to rest. A few minutes later, he announced that he had to throw up, so Annette quickly got a bowl for him. Annette decided to keep him home from nursery school and called the school and Lois, the mom who was driving that day, to let them know that Jonathan was not feeling well. Within fifteen minutes, however, Jonathan was up off the couch and announced that he felt fine and that he wanted to go to nursery school. Since he did not have a fever, Annette could see no reason to keep him home from school. She was able to reach Lois on her way out the door, so Jonathan went to nursery school after all.

For the next hour and a half, Annette was busy bathing, feeding, and playing with Stephanie. Annette put her down for her morning nap about ten o'clock. With the house quiet, Annette had time to think and reflect on the events of the last few days as she moved through the house, making beds and starting a load of laundry. Impulsively, she decided to call their pediatrician and ask her if she had any thoughts about Jonathan's headaches. Annette felt absolutely no panic—just parental concern that her child was complaining of headaches: Was it sinus? An eye problem? The doctor came on the telephone line and told Annette that she wanted Jonathan to go to the hospital at 1:00 P.M. for a CAT scan and that it was imperative that Jonathan not eat anything after breakfast. Annette quickly called the nursery school and was relieved that the children had not yet had snack time. She explained to the director that Jonathan was having a CAT scan that afternoon and that he was not to eat his snack. She then called their next-door neighbor, Debbie, to ask if she could baby-sit Stephanie and explained about Jonathan's CAT scan. It was then that Annette found out that Jonathan had commented to Debbie the day before, while Annette was at work, that his head hurt. Debbie had thought so little of it that she had forgotten to mention it to Annette when she picked the children up later in the day.

Annette made lunch for herself and Stephanie before Jonathan came home from nursery school. When he got home, she explained that their doctor wanted Jonathan to have a test at the hospital to determine why his head hurt. Annette still felt absolutely no panic or foreboding and did not question at all why a CAT scan was needed. She was so unconcerned that she did not even call Dan at work to let him know what was going on.

After bundling up Stephanie in her coat and mittens and dropping her off next door with Debbie, Annette and Jonathan drove to the local hospital just five minutes away. Jonathan was somewhat used to the hospital and the check-in procedure. At his fifteen-month check-up he was found to have a mild case of asthma and had gone for regular blood tests for the next couple of years. Annette had always stayed with him during his blood tests, talking calmly to him, and stroking his forehead as first he screamed and then whimpered with the discomfort. This time he was given an injection to sedate him for the CAT scan. After a half hour, he was no closer to sleep, so he was given another injection. He was given three injections in all, but he kept fighting sleep. He was then wheeled into the room with the CAT scanner . . . a huge machine . . . like a big doughnut . . . with a long, narrow bed that slid through the "doughnut." Jonathan was put on the long narrow bed and strapped down. Annette watched from the control room with the CAT technician. A patient must remain absolutely motionless for the CAT scan to be accurate. Jonathan, however, kept crying and would not lie still. Finally, Annette went into the room, pulled up a chair, rested Jonathan's head on her lap, stroked his forehead, and sang lullabies to him . . . He was soon asleep. Back in the control room, Annette watched the technician taking the various scans. She was fascinated with the equipment, the monitors, all the buttons and the switches, the pictures of Jonathan's brain appearing on the screens. Finally, the CAT scans were complete. Jonathan was sound asleep, so he was wheeled to a treatment room. Because by now it was after 5:00 P.M., Annette called Stephanie's baby-sitter to let her know that the CAT scan had taken much longer than anticipated.

As Annette was sitting in a chair next to Jonathan's bed, their pediatrician walked in. She made no eye contact with Annette but walked over to Jonathan's bed. *What a somber, serious gaze*, Annette thought, as the pediatrician looked down at Jonathan's sleeping, peaceful face. She looked up at Annette and said, "It's not good." Annette felt panic. The pediatrician said, "I want you to call your husband and ask him to come to the hospital." Stiffly, Annette walked to the nearby phone, sat down, and dialed the number. *I can't talk to him*, she thought, and suddenly her throat choked with unuttered sobs of fear. She went back to Jonathan's bedside and just stood there looking at him. *NO, NO, NO . . . Please, God, don't let there be anything wrong . . . NO!!* Annette saw the pediatrician on the phone talking to Dan but was unable to overhear her conversation.

For Dan, that phone discussion with the pediatrician was like being in the "twilight zone." He could not be hearing correctly . . . "Something tragically serious is wrong with Jonathan; you need to come to the hospital." Dan asked "Was there an accident?" The doctor said, "No." Dan was puzzled, frustrated . . . *What had happened today?* Dan beseeched the doctor to be straight with him . . . The feeling of being held in suspense was almost irritating . . . "If there was no accident, and I know that Jonathan is healthy, then what's the problem?" She finally told him. "A mass has been found on the CAT film." "What do you mean, a mass? What CAT film? What are you talking about?" . . . *There was nothing wrong with Jonathan . . . Annette would have called him if something serious had come up.* The doctor replied, "He was having some headaches." Dan mumbled, "I didn't even know anything about headaches." "Annette brought him in, and we did a CAT scan, and the mass is a brain tumor." Dan almost started arguing with the doctor: "How could that be? He seems so healthy. You mean Jonathan—my Jonathan?" Almost sternly, the doctor said, "It looks very serious, possibly terminal. Annette needs you at this time, and you need to come to the hospital."

Dan hung up the phone . . . numb . . . exhausted . . . feeling out of control . . . feeling as though his blood and energy were draining from his body. *Not my precious, adorable Jonathan.* In seconds he had crossed the room and was in the office of his good friend and cohort, Skip. Skip was a committed family man and father of three; he and Dan had had many conversations about their children over coffee, or while traveling together on business. Tears suddenly began pouring down Dan's face. Skip looked up in astonishment, then quickly stood up and put his arms around Dan as he wept. Dan was finally able to blurt out, "Jonathan has a brain tumor, and I have to go to the hospital." Skip was shocked, stunned, frozen, but reacted calmly for Dan's sake, "Now's the time to take care of Annette; be strong and rational. Don't worry about anything here. Just get to the hospital safely."

The forty-five-minute drive to the hospital was a blur as Dan's subconscious mind took over the familiar drive. As he approached the hospital, he felt a strong sense of approach-avoidance within him. He desperately felt compelled to be in there with Jonathan . . . but he was so scared, so scared . . . *God, help me!*

While Dan was driving to the hospital, Jonathan was moved up to the pediatric floor because he was still asleep. A nurse came into the room and commented on Jonathan's Cabbage Patch doll still by his side. It was one that Annette had made for him. Cabbage Patch dolls had hit the market big that year, and a store-bought doll was extremely hard to find. Annette told the nurse that he loved his doll and that he was getting another one for his fourth birthday, just eight days away. It was another handmade doll but made by a lady who made and sold the Cabbage Patch dolls. The conversation with the nurse was a welcome respite; Annette wanted the moments in the room with sleeping Jonathan to last forever . . . because for now everything was still okay.

Dan walked into the hospital in a daze. He felt out of place and uncomfortable; his only experience with medicine and with hospitals was with the birth of babies . . . Everything seemed in a vacuum, in slow motion . . . He was directed to Jonathan's room. Dan walked into the room . . . calmly but with haunted eyes. He looked down at his beautiful son sleeping peacefully. "Do you know what the problem is?" he asked Annette. "No," she said. He choked out the words, "It's a brain tumor." The words impaled themselves in Annette's heart . . . The dam of tears finally broke loose.

# 2

# The Tragic Prognosis

*Her piercing eyes* bore into Dan and Annette as though to verify that they were listening and comprehending, "It looks grave . . . It looks terminal . . . the tumor is so massive." Dan and Annette sat close together at a conference table; the pediatrician sat perpendicular to them. When she had closed the conference room door behind her, Dan had felt as though the tiny room were a prison cell and that the prison guard was about to hand down the sentence. The doctor's eyes kept staring at them as they both just sat there, numb and in shock. Dan tried to tell himself that he should be able to deal with this; he had just taught a session on stress management. Intellectually, he knew that he was in the "shock" stage, but emotionally he could not progress beyond that. "It is urgent that you talk with a neurosurgeon immediately." Dan and Annette never responded to the pediatrician—just kept staring at her as she talked. *What is a neurosurgeon? Guide us, doctor, we are at your mercy . . . Tell us what to do—you are the expert.* "I refer my patients to one of two neurosurgeons in the area. I have talked with one of them, and he can see you right away and wants you to be at the hospital tomorrow. Pack a suitcase; you may be there a while." *Yes, doctor, we will do as you say, we've only dealt with ear infections and asthma before. We know nothing about medicine and doctors and what we're supposed to do. We will go home and pack . . . Whatever you say.*

Back home, Dan dropped Annette and Jonathan off and went next door to get Stephanie. By now it was after 7:00 P.M., so Debbie was concerned as she answered the door. Dan stepped in and motioned to Bob, her husband, that he wanted to talk to him away from the kids. Bob led him to a bedroom, where Dan broke down crying and said, "Jonathan has a massive brain tumor; it looks terminal." Bob was speechless, visibly shaken, and never said a word while Dan calmed himself, collected Stephanie, and left.

Dan and Annette went through the evening never communicating with each other about the day's tragic events but instead making a concerted effort to maintain normalcy for the children the rest of the evening. They went through their usual routine ... made supper for the kids, let Jonathan and Stephanie play for a little while, read Jonathan a bedtime story, gave Stephanie her bedtime bottle. Dan and Annette explained to Jonathan that "there is a ball in your head that's making your head hurt. We have to go to the hospital tomorrow so they can get it out; otherwise the ball will grow bigger and make your head hurt even more."

Dan called his parents and broke the news to his mother. As he cried with her, he felt her pain, for she had lost a son eight years earlier, in December 1978, after just a five-month battle with leukemia. Dan and John had been five years apart and shared the same bedroom as they were growing up. The memory of his brother, John, was one reason that Dan had favored naming his firstborn son Jonathan. The death of John Lennon also came to Dan's mind, for John Lennon had been killed just days before Jonathan's birth. As a teenager, Dan had idolized the Beatles, particularly John Lennon, which was another reason he liked the name Jonathan. Dan was not a superstitious person, but he could not stop the irrational thought from repeating itself over and over in his mind that *the other two*

*Johns had died . . . one from cancer . . . the other just days before Jonathan was born . . . and they had both died in December . . . and this is December . . . and that has to mean that Jonathan is also going to die.* Later, with Jonathan and Stephanie in their beds, Dan lay in bed . . . praying . . . in a stupor . . . a daze . . . alone . . . waiting for the next day . . . praying some more . . . thinking of the deaths of his brother John and John Lennon . . . and having named his firstborn son after them both. . .

Annette's mind felt like a whirlwind; she could not yet think about the shocking news and what it meant for Jonathan. Her only thoughts focused on all the commitments she had to cancel for the rest of the week. A phone call to her boss's husband, "Please tell Carolyn that I won't be in tomorrow; Jonathan has a brain tumor and has to go to the hospital." A call to Lois, "I won't be able to drive to nursery school on Thursday; Jonathan has a brain tumor and has to go to the hospital tomorrow." A call to the president of one of her organizations, "I can't be at the meeting on Saturday; my son has a brain tumor and has to go to the hospital." A call to the prayer chain of the church's Women's Circle, "Please pray for Jonathan. He has a massive brain tumor and has to go to the hospital tomorrow." A call to Vickie, "We won't be at play group on Friday; Jonathan has a brain tumor and has to go to the hospital tomorrow." Finally a phone call to her parents, amazingly calm while breaking the bad news to them. As she made the phone calls, she was amazed at how calm she felt and how unemotionally she was able to relay the news. She could visualize the shock that the person at the other end of the line must be feeling as she broke the news of Jonathan's brain tumor to them. She felt as though she were in a movie, playing the part of a distraught mother trying to cope with a tragedy. She had to break off each call with a quick "good-bye" before the listener could say a word; she knew that she would break down if she began talking about the horrible news.

Now what has to be done? . . . Her mind still felt like a whirlwind, she was having difficulty focusing and concentrating; she packed a bag for Jonathan—a change of clothes, his Cabbage Patch doll, Matchbox cars, Transformers (small robot-like toys that "transformed" into cars or trucks), books, coloring books—and a bag for herself and Dan. *Okay, what else do I have to do? Get Stephanie's things ready for the baby-sitter . . . Empty the dishwasher . . . Go through the mail . . . Are there any bills to pay? . . . Periodically walk into Jonathan's room and just stare at him . . . Kiss his serene, sleeping face . . . Look in at Dan lying in bed with his eyes closed . . . Was he sleeping?* And throughout the whole evening she found that if she even so much as thought, *Why us?* her mind immediately responded with *Why* not *us? Tragedies happened to other people all the time; why are we immune?* The night passed too slowly . . . *Just can't settle down to sleep . . . Have to keep getting up to go into Jonathan's room and just look at him.* The night passed too quickly . . . Sooner and sooner daybreak was coming . . . *I can't cry. . . . This is so scary.*

During the drive to the hospital early the next morning as Dan flipped through the radio stations, he was haunted by John Lennon's "Imagine" on one of the stations; he quickly turned the radio off . . . thinking that his son would also die. Annette had the totally illogical thought of stopping at the mall on the way to the hospital so that Jonathan could have his annual "birthday" portrait taken . . . He would be four years old in just one week . . . and he might be dead by then. Neither Dan nor Annette talked of their private thoughts; the drive was silent. Jonathan sat in the back in his booster seat viewing the passing landscape.

The elevator ride from the parking garage to the hospital seemed interminable, creaking and stopping at every floor.

A well-dressed couple entered the elevator, talking of their newborn nephew they were going to visit. Dan listened with envy, with thoughts of escape. *I wish I were they . . . healthy . . . nothing wrong . . .* Guilt washed over him . . . *Maybe God is punishing us . . . There has to be a reason that God is doing this to Jonathan. Maybe we haven't been appreciative enough of what we already have. Maybe he's punishing us for not putting him first in our lives during college . . . when we didn't go to church regularly . . . Maybe we did things back then that he didn't like.* Thoughts of self-blame flashed through his heart like lightning bolts. *What have we done to our son?*

After checking in and settling themselves in Jonathan's room, the nurse stopped by and said that the doctor would be by soon to talk with them. Jonathan sat on his bed watching "Sesame Street" and coloring in a coloring book. Annette found herself just standing at the window, gazing out at the everyday, ordinary activities going on outside the confines of the hospital walls . . . *So many people don't even realize the pain and the emotions going on inside here . . . and before today, I never understood, either.* A couple of hours later, the doctor finally stopped by and introduced himself; he took Jonathan's CAT scans that Dan and Annette had brought along and said that he wanted to study the films before talking with them later in the day.

The next few hours of waiting were spent in the toy room. Jonathan's favorite game with Dan since infancy had been playing "three balls for a quarter." Jonathan would sit on top of the couch, laughing and shrieking with anticipation while Dan armed himself with a soft Nerf ball. Dan would exaggerate a wild pitch as the ball would fly through the air toward Jonathan. If the ball hit Jonathan, he would fall onto the couch laughing hysterically. Jonathan absolutely loved the game and almost every evening would beg Dan to play. The game that the two of them invented in the toy room was a variation of "three balls for a quarter." Dan built a tower from big cardboard "red brick" blocks, the kind often found in day-care centers and nursery schools. Jonathan giggled with glee as he tried to knock them down with a well-aimed throw of a soft ball. The scene was one of such innocence—a seemingly perfectly healthy child, laughing and playing with his parents in a room full of toys. The parents tried so hard to make this a happy day for Jonathan, before he had to experience the inevitable pain and suffering that were sure to come.

The toy room was theirs alone . . . theirs to pretend that all was right with their son . . . theirs to savor the time spent playing with their son. Then their minister arrived, bringing reality with him as he walked in with a seriousness that told Dan and Annette that he fully understood the gravity of Jonathan's diagnosis. He held out his arms to Annette and seemed surprised that she did not fall into them, hysterical with grief. He asked if he could pray with them. Dan and Annette listened in disbelief as the minister intoned, ". . . and be with this couple and give them courage even if this child should die." "Wait a minute," Dan burst out, "that's not my prayer. I'm not praying for that. I am praying to God that he save my child." The minister tried to convince Dan and Annette that "we must accept reality; children do die, and Jonathan may die." "NO!" Dan felt a burst of fury and kicked a block across the room. "No! I believe that God answers prayers if it's his will, and I am praying that he save my child." Annette could not believe that her minister had come to the hospital to provide this sort of "comfort" for them . . . *Why am I even listening to this? . . . Time is so precious with Jonathan* . . . She left Dan and returned to Jonathan's side to join in his play. Dan felt himself moving out of the "shock" stage and felt a spurt of a fighting spirit within him . . . *Why am I debating theology at a time like this when my wife and child need me?* Dan grew increasingly impatient. Finally, he thanked the minister for coming, and the visit ended.

Reality later intruded again into the serenity of the toy room when a nurse came in and asked Dan and Annette to go to the conference room where the doctor was waiting to talk with them. He commented that he would not have ordered a CAT scan as had the pediatrician, based on just a few minor headaches. In fact, the pediatrician would later say that she did not know what had led her to order a CAT scan. The neurosurgeon seemed precise and mechanical, almost as though he were describing an engineering process, forgetting that he was talking to the distraught parents of a young child as he explained the procedure he was proposing to perform on Jonathan the next day. The visualization of "drilling and sawing his skull open" tore into Dan's gut with sickening pain. These procedures used tools that should be used for metal and wood, not for children! Annette could not keep her eyes off the section on the consent form that listed possible complications: "paralysis, death." The doctor stressed the urgency of performing surgery immediately, stating that he didn't know how fast the tumor was growing; that the more it grew, the more chance there would be of permanent brain damage or death; that the tumor was massive; that he wasn't optimistic; that he would try to take as much of the tumor out as possible; that after the surgery he would better know what kind of tumor it was; and that Jonathan would most likely have permanent coordination problems, since the tumor was in the cerebellum (the coordination part of the brain). Terrible thought that it was, Annette found herself half-wishing that if Jonathan were to end up with severe physical handicaps that he would die instead.

As the doctor awaited their signatures, Dan and Annette

seemed to come to their senses and began asking the doctor questions: "What would you do if this were your son?" . . . "Go ahead and perform the surgery tomorrow; we don't know what kind of tumor Jonathan has or how fast it will grow." Dan emphasized to the doctor that "we want the very best care for our child and will go anywhere in the country to get it . . . We can afford it, plus we have one hundred percent insurance." The doctor said his hospital's equipment was as up-to-date as any hospital's in the country. The doctor was asked how many of this type of surgery he did. He responded by quoting a statistic: "There are 'x' number of neurosurgeons in the country and 'x' number of brain tumor surgeries a year, so that means that no surgeon does more than two or three a year," and that he personally saw a couple of similar cases a year. The doctor was asked if there were any doctors who were better at this type of surgery. He responded that he had trained in New York with the team of doctors who had performed surgery on the Shah of Iran.

Dan and Annette felt they were asking intelligent questions, but unfortunately and unknowingly they were caught up in the "false trust syndrome," meaning that they still had total faith in the medical system and in doctors. It absolutely never crossed their minds that they should request or seek a second opinion. None of their family or friends or co-workers ever suggested to them that they might consider getting a second opinion. Dan and Annette believed the doctor's answers to their questions, and they believed his sense of urgency to perform surgery. They signed the consent form. The surgery was scheduled for the next morning.

The very worst part of that day for Dan was returning to the toy room and resuming play with Jonathan. All he could think of was that the next day the surgeon was going to split his young son's head open . . . That thought brought non-

ending, wrenching heartache and pain. He could not stop
blaming himself . . . *Why am I letting this happen to my child?*
The guilt he felt was immense. When Annette brought
Jonathan back to his room to rest, Dan stayed in the toy
room and prayed and prayed to God to please save his son.

As Annette sat next to Jonathan's bed, watching Sesame
Street with him, her dear friend Darla walked into the room.
Immediately, all Annette's tears that had been unshed for
the last twenty-four hours unleashed themselves, and as she
finally sobbed and sobbed, Darla left the room until the tears
ran dry. Darla and Annette had worked together at Davis
College since Annette began there five years earlier. They
were close friends before Jonathan's birth and remained very
close friends afterward, even when Annette had taken a
leave to earn her M.B.A. degree. Darla had been one of the
first people to visit both Jonathan and Stephanie after their
births and had remained intimately involved in their growing
up. Darla had brought M&Ms for Jonathan—his favorite
candy. Annette explained to Darla everything that had
happened and the surgery the next day. Dan returned to the
room, and they all discussed the minister's visit and the
debate he had engendered. Darla prayed with them before
she left. Dan also left soon after, to spend the night at home
with Stephanie.

That evening Dan was thankful that Stephanie was
cheerful, ate well, and fell asleep early. A family friend,
Diana, called, expressing her sympathy at the news. Dan
would not stop talking. Diana asked several times if Dan
wanted her and her husband Tom to come over; he kept
saying no but could not stop talking. He did not want to be
alone, yet he did not want people . . . but he finally said
good-bye to her. He was reluctant to call family, friends . . .
not wanting to impose his pain and suffering on them . . . not
realizing that many people *want* to help in times of

emotional need. He spent the night crying . . . every part of
his body in pain, nerves tingling . . . sitting in bed drinking
beer to dull the pain . . . eventually making a path from bed
to bathroom to refrigerator for another beer and back to bed
. . . continuing to cry in anguish. The night was as restless
and unsettled as Dan; the wind blew against the windows and
through the trees as a winter storm moved into the area.

Annette spent the night on a cot in Jonathan's room. A
resident came and took Jonathan's H&P (history and
physical); someone else came in and took blood from
Jonathan. Poor little guy . . . so brave . . . never questioning
his parents about what was going on. Annette asked the
resident if he could give her something to help her relax; he
said he was not allowed to prescribe medication for the
parents. She realized then that hospitals do not really
concern themselves with the parents' emotional state. She
settled Jonathan into bed, read him a couple of stories, and
lay down with him until he fell asleep. She tried to read . . .
tried to watch TV . . . and eventually fell into a fitful sleep.

As Annette waited for Dan to arrive the next morning,
she again gazed out the window at the activity below. Snow
had fallen during the night, and she imagined herself at
home . . . bundling Jonathan into his snowsuit, preparing
him for nursery school . . . taking Stephanie and Jonathan
later in the day for a walk around the block, pulling them on
their sled. She felt extremely sad that life had changed so
dreadfully for Jonathan and the family.

The thought uppermost in Dan's mind during his drive
to the hospital was concern that the neurosurgeon was
feeling fine and alert. Being sports-minded, Dan knew that
top performance was greatly dependent on physical and
mental well-being. In fact, the first question he asked the
doctor at the hospital was, "How are you feeling today?" The
doctor looked at him in surprise and said, "Oh, I'm fine."

On impulse, in the room with Jonathan, Dan decided to give Jonathan a little "test"—more for peace of mind for Dan, so that he would know after the surgery whether or not Jonathan had suffered any cognitive brain damage. Dan asked Jonathan to show him how to "transform" a particularly difficult Transformer, which required excellent eye-hand coordination as well as memory of having done it before. Dan also told Jonathan that he would get him a Voltron Lion for his birthday, a toy that Jonathan had been particularly wanting. After surgery, Dan would ask Jonathan to again "transform" the Transformer and to remember what special toy he would be getting for his birthday. Dan explained to Jonathan that the surgery was not going to hurt, because the doctor would put a mask on his face that would make him fall asleep, and that when he woke up, the "ball" would be out of his head. Jonathan's main concern, however, as he was being wheeled down the hall toward the operating room was, "Just don't let them see my butt." Oh, the innocence of a child!

Dan and Annette watched in silence as Jonathan was wheeled through the operating room doors. "We'll see you later, Jonathan!" As they walked back down the hallway toward Jonathan's room, there was Carolyn, Annette's boss, getting off the elevator. Again, pent-up emotion and tears seemed to flow out of Annette as she let herself be enveloped in Carolyn's warm, secure embrace. Carolyn waited with Dan and Annette in the surgery waiting room while they explained to her everything the doctor had told them the day before. The wait in that room was interminable as the minutes and hours ticked by slowly. Dan and Annette were never alone for long, as a steady stream of Annette's fellow workers, in groups of two or three, came for a short time and then left. Annette would find out later that her co-workers were determined that Dan and Annette would not be left alone and had purposely timed everyone's visits to make sure that someone was always there.

Throughout the day, Dan purposely allowed himself to feel the pain of grief and fear and terror . . . He wanted to feel the same pain that his child was feeling . . . to be able to trade places with his child. Dan was entering the "bargaining" stage and wanting to make deals with God. The prayers of the minister who had prayed for Jonathan with the assumption of his probable death still haunted the minds of Dan and Annette. *Perhaps the minister was right*, thought Dan. Confusion set in for them. Then someone announced to Dan and Annette that Pat Robertson had been praying on the CBN "700 Club" that God would touch Jonathan with his holy power and that Jonathan would be healed. This message was very inspirational for Dan and Annette and assured them that they were right to pray for healing. Other people told them of prayer chains all around the country who were praying for Jonathan. Some late-afternoon visitors brought a sense of spiritual healing into the room. Two of Annette's co-workers and their husbands, one of them a minister, had come by. The six of them sat in a circle, holding hands, feeling the presence of God in their midst as a prayer was lifted up to God for the healing of Jonathan . . . for a miracle.

Shortly thereafter, about six hours after Jonathan had been wheeled through the operating room doors, the surgery was over. A nurse escorted Dan and Annette to a surgical anteroom where the neurosurgeon was waiting for them. Dan was prepared for good news, but one look at the doctor's discouraged face and downcast eyes pierced his optimism. The doctor's nonverbals told Dan that the surgery must not have gone well. The doctor kept repeating, "It just wasn't what I expected." "What do you mean?" Dan insisted. "Is that good or bad?" The doctor explained—"I took as much out as I could, but I had to stop when I couldn't tell what was good tissue and what was bad tissue. There was no line of demarcation. I really took my time, but I had to stop. There is tumor on the brain stem, and it's too risky to operate there." All Annette cared about was that Jonathan was alive; she was not hearing any of the bad news but just the doctor saying that he had resected as much as he could and had not taken any good brain tissue . . . which to her meant there was probably no brain damage. For her, at that point, the news was good. For Dan, however, the news was ambiguous but terrible—there was still tumor left.

Dan and Annette were brought to the room next to Jonathan's, where they would be able to spend the night since the pediatric floor was fairly empty. As they waited for Jonathan to return from the recovery room, the neurosurgeon stopped by. He told them that Jonathan would be in Intensive Care for several hours. He repeated again that the tumor "wasn't what I expected, but I've done some reading. Basically, the rest of his tumor is inoperable; operating on the brain stem is too risky. Right now some hospitals are experimenting with CAT-guided laser techniques, but that's probably a couple of years away yet. Surgically, nothing more can be done for Jonathan. So my advice to you is to live each day as his last." "What do you mean?" Dan wanted to know. "What are you saying?" The doctor explained that "in this situation, it's just a matter of time. We cannot operate any more on Jonathan's tumor. And at his young age, radiation and chemotherapy are done only when he's getting really bad. Even then, it would only be buying time, as the tumor would not be completely eradicated. So live each day as his last." Dan demanded to know, "What does that mean? How *many* days?" The doctor's devastating reply was, "Maybe a couple of months, maybe a couple of years."

# 3

# Hitting Bottom—God Where Are You?

*Dan and Annette looked at the doctor in shock.* When he left, they each fell onto a bed and broke into heartbreaking, excruciatingly painful wails of anguish. Dan felt cold, empty, abandoned, lonely, helpless, for indeed the death sentence had been handed down. He felt déja vu as he remembered his brother John's slow, tortured death through five months of chemotherapy . . . the hair loss, the gagging, and throwing up the huge pills he had to swallow . . . his mother searching through the vomit to regain the pill . . . the growing weakness . . . constantly spitting into a bucket . . . so pale and sickly, the constant discomfort and pain . . . his mother's heart breaking as she nursed her son to his death. Dan could not bear the thought of such a grotesque death for his little boy.

Dan knew now that he truly needed God, and he came to the only conclusion that he could accept—to have God just take Jonathan rather than put him through such pain and misery. As he lay on the bed sobbing in grief, Dan remembered something that his mother had said a long time after his brother's death: "A child is really God's child; our job as parents is to be that child's guardian throughout his life. When God decides to take back his child, we must be able to let that child go; otherwise, we die with that child.

41

Only if we can let that child return to God, will we ourselves be able to go on with life." In his grief, Dan decided that he was not going to die with his child but that he was placing Jonathan in God's hands. Peace and strength slowly began to flow into Dan.

As Annette lay on the bed, she let the gut-wrenching sobs rip through her heart and body. She wept and wept with the pain that she would never see Jonathan grow up . . . never see him off on his first day of school . . . never watch him play Little League . . . never see him mature as a teenager and have girlfriends . . . never see him become a husband and father. She wept for all the years of raising him through infancy and toddlerhood, all the good times, all the trying times, only to have it all end . . . and just when he had become such a delightful, independent little boy. All those months of pregnancy during which she had been so careful . . . no alcohol . . . lots of fruits and vegetables . . . all in vain. As Annette immersed herself in grief, she felt that God was helping her see into the future . . . She could see herself . . . playing with Stephanie . . . talking about memories of Jonathan . . . returning to work . . . She knew that she would go through immense pain as she grieved for Jonathan, but she also somehow knew that God would enable her eventually to return to the mainstream of life and that she would never forget Jonathan but would be always thankful for the few short years with him. Even while weeping over the dreadful prognosis given to them by the neurosurgeon, Annette knew that God would want her to continue loving and enjoying Jonathan in his remaining time on earth and that he would stand beside her in her grief.

Yet the tears continued to flow. One of Annette's coworkers came to visit, but Dan went out into the hall to tell her the bad prognosis and that Annette was in no condition to see visitors. Annette finally cried herself into exhaustion and fell into a deep, deep sleep. Dan left her there to sleep and went into Jonathan's room next door, stationing himself in a chair to await Jonathan's return from the recovery room. He was startled by a big, burly orderly pushing Jonathan's bed into the room. Still sleeping, the little boy's head was wrapped in a big bandage, an IV went into his arm, a monitor bleep-bleeped steadily. Dan forced himself to stay awake all night, treasuring every moment with Jonathan, asking the results of his vital signs as the nurses came in regularly. He wanted to know every detail of his son's condition as if every moment of Jonathan's life depended on his father's taking care of him. Throughout the long night Dan felt a determination growing slowly in him, felt himself growing stronger, and realized that *if I am putting Jonathan in God's hands, I have to take care of my son and do whatever I can do to help save his life.*

As daybreak came and the workers began changing shifts and duties, Dan struggled to stay awake. Annette came into Jonathan's room, calm with the knowledge that her role was to continue loving and enjoying Jonathan's time here on earth. When Jonathan finally awoke, he looked so good, so alert. With anxiety, Dan walked to Jonathan's bedside and knelt down and whispered in his ear, "Do you remember what I'm going to get you for your birthday, Jonathan?" Jonathan seemed to ponder too long . . . *Oh, no*, Dan thought . . . but then, with his voice hoarse from the anesthesia tube, Jonathan whispered, "A Voltron Lion." "Oh, Jonathan," Dan said and hugged him with tears of joy.

Their time together was interrupted by the neurosurgeon's walking into the room. The doctor watched in amazement as Jonathan put together the Transformer that Dan had been saving for this moment. The doctor asked for the toy and after several tries himself, admitted defeat. It was then that Dan felt the first niggling of doubt, *Wait a minute, maybe this doctor's not a god—he may be fallible*, but immediately he told himself that he was being unfair.

Later that morning, the doctor again returned to the room, this time to report that he had been doing some more research on Jonathan's tumor and to give them the results of the preliminary pathology report. The tumor was a Grade 1, the slowest-growing of four possible grades, Grade 4 being the most malignant and the fastest-growing. The doctor seemed pleased to report that he was revising his prognosis because the tumor was the slow-growing Grade 1 type. He now felt encouraged that perhaps Jonathan would be able to live at least three to five years instead of possibly just a few months and that by that time, technology may have advanced. The doctor stressed again, though, that the problem with Jonathan's tumor was not the grade but the location: "We just cannot operate on the brain stem."

Heartbreaking though the prognosis still was, it was getting better! Annette called the banquet hall at which her co-workers were having their annual Christmas luncheon and relayed the improved prognosis. She would later be told that the mood at the luncheon prior to her call had been bleak and sad as everyone shared in the terrible prognosis from the evening before. After her phone call, the mood became merry and joyous as befitted a Christmas celebration. That afternoon, the seriousness of the situation was further dispelled, and Dan and Annette smiled for the first time. Coming down the hall, incongruous with death and illness, were two little, white-haired, grandmotherly women in Gray Lady volunteer uniforms. They came into the room, greeted Dan and Annette, and said, "We have been praying so hard for your son; he's so important to us."

Even though Jonathan looked great, the gravity of his condition was brought home many times throughout his week-long hospital stay. The day after surgery he felt the back of his head, which was still bandaged, and announced that he did not want anyone to see his head. Annette bought him a large-size man's hat that Jonathan wore everywhere for the next several weeks as the surgical site healed. Friends and relatives came to visit Jonathan, bringing him gifts and marveling at how wonderful he looked. Annette empathized with the visitors, who were surely inwardly recoiling in horror at the thought of this beautiful little boy having only years left to live. Some friends would not even come upstairs to Jonathan's room, so Annette had to go down to the lobby to talk with them. A couple of people could not even bring themselves to go to the hospital but relayed their messages through other friends. Dan and Annette felt somehow betrayed by these people and realized then how important it is for people to confront their friends' grief and suffering and to provide much-needed support. Annette forced herself to be cheerful and upbeat during these visits because she did not want people's pity.

One of Dan's most comforting visits was from Rick, a friend from his office. Rick possessed a deep faith in God and was genuine and sincere. When he visited Dan, he was soft-spoken and slow to speak, searching for the right words. As he and Dan held on to each other, the tears in Rick's eyes told Dan that Rick understood and that no more words were necessary.

Walking through the halls of the pediatric floor, carrying Jonathan, would bring Dan face-to-face with the seriousness of Jonathan's condition. Other parents would be walking with their children, trailing IV tubes. After several conversations with different parents, Dan realized that the other pediatric cases were mainly hernia operations, pneumonia, and tonsillectomies. When Dan would tell the other parents that his son had just had brain surgery, the other parents would stop in shock, mumble a few words, and quickly leave with their small children—unable to deal with such a grave condition. Dan realized then that most parents, unless they are faced with the same heartbreak, cannot relate to parents of terminally ill children.

Dan stayed at the hospital days and nights for that week and took over the daily care of Jonathan, bathing him, playing with him, bringing him to the doctor to have his wound aspirated (excess fluid drained from the surgical site), and comforting Jonathan through the discomfort. Annette went home every night to be with Stephanie. Stephanie stayed with two or three different baby-sitters every day as the women of the church's Women's Circle took over the responsibility of providing care for Stephanie. Annette was thankful that Stephanie, only eight-and-a-half-months old, coped so well with the ever-changing flow of homes she was brought into daily; she adjusted easily into each family's routine as she "blossomed" and "entertained" her hosts; she truly loved being around people. Nightly, a meal was brought over by a compassionate neighbor or friend because Annette had already lost several pounds; the last thing on her mind when in the hospital with Jonathan was the need to eat.

Alone, away from Jonathan and the hospital routine, Annette felt the need to talk with faraway friends and share the events of the last week but never could bring herself to call anyone and relay such shocking news to people over the phone. One night Dan called her and told her that the doctor was worried about hydrocephalus, swelling of the brain, and the possibility of shunts and tubes. *No, I can't handle any more*, she cried to herself. She found herself calling Jan, a friend from play group, and breaking down in tears over the phone; Jan immediately came over and sat with Annette on the couch, holding her in her arms as Annette cried tears that had been pent up for several days.

"How much more do we have to deal with? I can't take any more!" cried Annette. Sometimes, it all seemed like a nightmare from which they couldn't wake up.

Both Annette and Jonathan celebrated their birthdays one day apart in the hospital with cakes made by one of Annette's co-workers. Jonathan celebrated his fourth birthday in the hospital's toy room, surrounded by presents. The neurosurgeon stopped by to offer his congratulations, as did the rest of the pediatric floor staff. Stephanie came to visit that day, carrying a huge Christmas teddy bear for Jonathan; she and Jonathan were ecstatic with glee when they saw each other.

One afternoon while Dan and Annette were in the toy room with Jonathan, an oncologist walked in, introduced herself, and sat down on the floor next to them. She said that their neurosurgeon had asked her to come to the hospital to discuss Jonathan's case. Her conclusion was that chemotherapy was not a viable option right now; that chemo was not the treatment of choice for this type of tumor in children; and that chemo would most likely be of no benefit to Jonathan. With that short summation of Jonathan, she left the room. Annette and Dan were left somewhat open-mouthed, as the visit had been totally unexpected and seemed so unprofessional.

Jonathan was allowed to return home after ten days in the hospital; the neighborhood children ran over to welcome him as the car pulled into the driveway. Except for his hat, he was fully recovered from the surgery and had absolutely no adverse results. Both Dan and Annette returned to work, Stephanie resumed her normal routine, and Jonathan went back to nursery school. Annette went with him the first day because she was concerned about the other children's reaction to Jonathan's hat. She sat with the children in their circle as they came into the room. She was surprised that the

children treated Jonathan as usual and did not even comment on his absence or his hat. Jonathan had his postponed
birthday party with his nursery school and neighborhood
friends and frolicked and gamboled with the rest of the little
boys. He looked and acted so normal that it was easy to
forget, momentarily, the reality. In retrospect, Annette and
Dan were amazed that even though the prognosis was still
terrible, they were able to resume a fairly normal life. They
felt as though dealing with the "death sentence" could be
temporarily put on hold. In the Christmas letter that
Annette wrote later that month to friends and relatives, she
said, "Dan and I did remarkably well. Within two days after
surgery, there were no more tears. We just took one step at
a time, adjusted to that, and moved on. The whole thing was
incredibly painful, but we had to cope—there was no choice.
We were amazed at the inner strength a person has when
facing this."

Christmas pictures in the photo album show joy and
laughter and Jonathan full of smiles opening his Christmas
presents—but always wearing his hat to cover his wound. At
Dan's family get-together, his mother had given all the
grandchildren hats so that Jonathan would fit right in.

Jonathan looked great but still had a tumor in his head,
and that reality kept forcing itself to the surface of Dan's and
Annette's lives even as they tried to make life as normal as
possible for Jonathan and Stephanie. The long winter days of
January and February grew increasingly difficult. Annette
found that she could not sleep, because it was then that the
stark reality of Jonathan's prognosis would hit her heart.
Once the children were in bed at 9:00, she needed to find
something to occupy her mind and turned to redecorating
the house—going from room to room, wallpapering, paint-
ing, tearing down paneling, staining trim and wainscoting.
Years later she would realize that to cope with Jonathan's

situation, she had needed to feel some sort of control, and the decorating had provided her with at least one area of total control in her life. In addition, by keeping her mind and body totally occupied nightly from 9:00 P.M. to 2:00 A.M., she was able to sink into an immediate, deep sleep and be refreshed every morning at 7:00 to begin the new day.

Dan found himself going through those days unable to concentrate at home and at work; his whole life became preoccupied with Jonathan's tumor; he felt increasingly helpless but could feel determination and rationality slowly beginning to build in him.

The most difficult part of those months was waiting for the monthly CAT scans Jonathan had at the hospital. Jonathan had to have an injection of dye each time, often necessitating several tries before finding a vein in his arm, and he would have to lie completely still for the half hour or so it took to complete the CAT scans. He always got to pick out a toy at Toys R Us on the way back home. For Dan and Annette, the anticipation, the not knowing, the tension were extremely stressful. After each session the neurosurgeon would show them the CAT scan, point to a small black hole, and announce that the tumor had not grown. He was always ambiguous, though, and would talk about surgical scarring and edema and not being able to exactly tell where the tumor was. He had once mentioned that he had an engineering background, and since Dan also had a technical background, they would often talk "shop." The doctor would explain why, surgically, Jonathan's tumor was basically inoperable—that the good tissue could not be delineated from the bad tissue—and that operating on and near the brain stem was extremely risky.

What Dan and Annette did not then know, however, was that the small black hole to which the neurosurgeon kept pointing was actually just the small portion of tumor that had been resected. During those months, they were always led to believe that the small black hole was the residual tumor, the tumor that the doctor had not been able to remove. Not knowing that important, crucial fact resulted in Annette's never realizing the true implications of the seriousness of Jonathan's condition. Her perception of Jonathan's just having a small tumor left that was not growing and that could somehow be removed if it did someday grow, frustrated Dan immensely. He felt that she was blocking out the seriousness of the situation, and he could not get her to discuss options. Dan would get angry with Annette and at her failure to face reality; he felt that she was "checking out." Annette felt that Dan was over-reacting. To her, Jonathan looked and acted fairly normal; ergo, he was fine. Other than the CAT scans, Jonathan was leading a perfectly normal four-year-old life, attending nursery school, and playing with his toys and friends. He had only minor, infrequent headaches and was showing no new symptoms.

During their visits with the neurosurgeon, Dan would intensely question him and become frustrated at his lack of answers; he began calling him "Dr. I-Don't-Know." Dan began asking that they be sent for a second opinion and emphasized again that they wanted to go to the best doctor and facility anywhere in the world. The neurosurgeon continued to insist that he and his hospital were as good as anyone or anyplace else and that no one operated on many brain tumors. Finally, the doctor relented and agreed to send Jonathan's records to a nationally renowned clinic at which a neurosurgeon was performing experimental surgery with computer-guided laser resection of tumors. Their doctor felt that this clinic was on the "cutting edge" of technology in resecting brain tumors, that the computer-guided laser surgery was a breakthrough, and that the ultimately tough cases went to this clinic. The impression given to Dan and

Annette was that this doctor was the number-one doctor in the world and that to get an opinion from him would negate the need to go anywhere else. The next couple of weeks were ones of anticipation and stress and *hope* as Dan and Annette eagerly awaited this clinic's response. Then, on a Saturday evening in early March, the neurosurgeon called. He had received a letter from the doctor at the nationally renowned clinic, and he summarized the letter to them over the phone. The words seared and imprinted themselves forever into the memories of Dan and Annette. "I could give this patient no guarantee that making a bigger hole in this tumor would be useful to him in the long run." For Dan, the world stopped; he knew he would always remember the moment in time when he was upstairs in the study and took the phone call from the neurosurgeon—just as so many people can forever remember the exact moment in time when they learned of President Kennedy's assassination in 1964. Reality hit, all hope was gone. Jonathan's one last chance at life was dashed. Feeling as though they had been dealt the final blow, Dan and Annette finally hit bottom. "God, where are you!" they cried.

# 4

# We're Not Giving Up

*The rest of the weekend passed in a daze* as both Dan and Annette tried to absorb the horrible fact that there was no hope . . . that they would lose their firstborn, precious little boy in a few years. How would he die? Would it be sudden? In his sleep? In his play? Would it be slow and painful? Would it begin by Jonathan's coordination being affected . . . falling a lot, running awkwardly . . . finally being unable to walk? What would they tell Jonathan? How would the neighbors and his playmates react? Would he finally be totally bedridden? Would other parts of his body start being affected . . . his speech, his hearing, his memory? *Oh, God, we're not strong enough! Give us strength.* Bouncing back and forth in their minds, occupying their thoughts, crowding everything else into the far recesses, were pleas to God: *We prayed! . . . We bargained! . . . We tried as hard as we could!*

Their subconscious minds taking over, both Dan and Annette went through the next week feeling lost in a fog, almost in a hypnotic state, with sleepless nights and drowsy days. Dan had hallucinating dreams of being in a foreign country, not speaking the language, lost, totally at the mercy of fate. He dreamed of being attacked and unable to scream, of feeling totally helpless. *God, why have you let us down? . . . Your son's going to die*, bleeped across his mind constantly, as well as haunting images of Jonathan's death and the horrible years ahead.

Both had difficulty focusing on day-to-day responsibilities and activities. They felt alone, as if God were not there. Once Dan found himself miles past his interstate exit on his way to work. Another day, while flying on a business trip, he was surprised to find himself already in the city of his destination; he had been so absorbed with thoughts of Jonathan that he hadn't even noticed the descent. One Sunday at church they were startled as they looked up and noticed people already leaving the sanctuary; how long had the service been over? Dan's friends and acquaintances would comment that he seemed distracted as he did his work. Yet how could he explain that dealing with the company's productivity concerns seemed so unimportant compared with the life of his son? Annette still felt as though she were in a nightmare from which she couldn't wake up. She withdrew to her desk at work; she couldn't face talking to people over lunch and coffee. She had a hard time talking about current events in her economics class; she could not find the enthusiasm and interest to care about what was happening in the world. Only Jonathan mattered. Only his brain tumor mattered.

The normal, happy feelings they once had were gone; instead they felt numbness, despair, and depression. Both grew thinner as they lost their desire for food. To make matters worse, Dan was regularly visiting a couple and their little girl who was also stricken with a terminal brain tumor. This little girl lived in a nearby small town and had been diagnosed with a brain tumor the same day and in the same hospital as Jonathan—the sheer coincidence created an aura of shock that hung over the hospital and their town for days. On each visit Dan could see the impending reality of her inevitable death. She was so pale and thin but so pretty with her blond hair and innocence. Her closeness to death became unbearable as he imagined his child in the same condition. He watched in deep sorrow and shared the pain and suffering with the parents. Soon he and Annette mourned her death at her funeral and felt guilty that their son was still alive and this little girl wasn't. The thought and reality that Jonathan would follow in her footsteps was devastating to them.

Friends and family tried to offer their own words of comfort, some of which Dan and Annette could not and would not accept. "Everything will be okay." (How do you know?) "God only gives us what we can handle." (*No*, we are no stronger than anyone else.) "God must have some reason that we don't know about." (*No*, he would not do this to a child for a reason or for a purpose—God is not a mean and cruel God.) "We're praying for a miracle." (What if God doesn't provide us a miracle, does that mean there is no God, that we're unworthy of a miracle?) The book that finally provided Annette with the most comfort and sense to the whole situation was *When Bad Things Happen to Good People* by Harold Kushner.[1] Bad things do happen to people . . . for no reason. They are just a part of life. Jonathan's brain tumor did not mean that God was punishing Dan and Annette, that he was punishing Jonathan, or that he had a "reason" for making such a small child suffer so much.

During this time, Annette began attending a cancer support group at the local hospital. Looking at and listening to the other people, all adult cancer patients, made Annette inordinately sad. They looked terrible—pale, one with a tracheotomy, another with hair loss—yet they were so positive and full of life. Didn't they know they were going to be dying soon? *Am I going to someday be like that*, thought Annette, *with a son who looks terrible to everyone else, but I'm*

---

Harold S. Kushner, *When Bad Things Happen to Good People*, Avon Books, New York, New York 10019, 1981.

*going to be prattling on at how well his treatment is going?* After two meetings, she decided that the meetings were making her feel worse, not better.

Dan spent many sleepless nights looking through the photo albums . . . reliving Jonathan's birth, his infancy, his toddlerhood. He would walk into Jonathan's room and gaze at his sleeping son and regularly find himself pacing back and forth from the family room into Jonathan's room. At Jonathan's bedtime, Dan would often sit with Jonathan and talk with him or read him a book; those moments were so precious. Still, during this time of despair, Dan would continue to pray for guidance. However, nothing was happening, only the constant pain and suffering.

Then one restless evening as Jonathan lay trying to sleep but suffering from yet another headache, he looked up and asked his father, "If the hospital got the ball out, why does my head still hurt?" Dan's heart sank . . . *Oh, my son, how do I tell you?* Dan put his arms around Jonathan and told him, "Sometimes when a person has a ball in his head, it's in a spot that's hard to get out. The doctor got part of the ball out, but there's still some left and that's why your head still hurts." Jonathan looked so sad, so worried. "Does that mean my head will always hurt, even when I'm a grownup?" Dan wanted to cry . . . *Oh, if you could only live to be a grownup.* Holding back the tears, he hugged Jonathan and told him, "You see, Jonathan, the doctors say they can't do anything more."

Jonathan sat up, turned to face Dan, tilted his baby-cheeked face upward, focused his big hazel eyes with an unflinching gaze into Dan's eyes, and said with the utmost sincerity and innocence to his hero, his daddy: "Daddy, you can help me. Daddy, you can do anything; I know you can."

Dan was startled by his little boy's response. He felt as though a bolt of lightning had shot through his body. He remembered the words of Pat Robertson praying for Jonathan's healing. He felt the power of the Holy Spirit building through his limbs, through his mind, through his heart, building more and more. *Why not?* Dan wondered. *I solve business problems; why can't I solve this one? I cannot let my son down; he is counting on me; he believes in me. I can't sit by and watch him die while I drown in my sorrow and self-pity. I must find a way to save his life. The hell with the doctors!* He bent over, grabbed Jonathan in a big bear hug, squeezed him tightly, and with a choked voice told his little boy, "Thank you, Jonathan. I love you; now go to sleep. We'll find a way to get that ball out of your head!" *And thank you, Lord; it's time for me to get to work!*

He spent the rest of the night charged with energy and determination. He felt as though he were at battle with the tumor; he was determined to be the victor over this disease. He felt alive again, ready to face life. He now had a mission—to save Jonathan, his little son who was counting on him. He wrote down notes and thoughts on sheets and sheets of paper. He finally mapped out an action plan and strategy and felt that God was guiding him. Before he left for work the next day, he told Annette, "We're going to fight; we're going to save Jonathan's life!" She looked at him in confusion, incomprehension. *What is he talking about?*

Back at the office, charged and energetic, he began putting his strategy into motion. He told all his co-workers that he was determined to find an answer to Jonathan's problem. He would preface every business meeting or consulting assignment contact with "My son has a brain tumor. If you know or hear of anything, please let me know." If he came into contact with a person who was a doctor or who had a friend or a relative who was a doctor, he would talk to that physician, gleaning all that doctor's knowledge about brain tumors. He could almost feel neighbors and friends thinking, "This poor father has gone mad; he's so desperate, he just can't accept reality." He began an intense study of the medical literature by reading everything he could about brain tumors, about astrocytoma brain tumors, about tumors in the cerebellum, about tumors in children, about diagnostic options and treatment plans, and about the prognosis predictions. He went to a nearby medical college library and copied dozens of pages from medical books. He visited bookstores, going to bookstores instead of restaurants on his business trips, buying any book that dealt with tumors, brain tumors, and cancer. He intensely studied macrobiotics; he went with a co-worker to a health-food nutritionist from Syria who tried to convince him that a regimen of herbs and certain combinations of health foods would help shrink Jonathan's tumor. He read that fish can cause brain tumors, and knowing that fish sticks had been one of Jonathan's favorite foods since infancy, Dan insisted that Annette prepare different meals. They began eating food recommended in the macrobiotics book because the book related true examples of people cured just because of a change in diet. The battle against Jonathan's brain tumor became an obsession with Dan.

Annette continued to frustrate Dan immensely. She listened with interest to his findings, his research, his theories, his determination to find a cure for Jonathan. Yet, Dan called her an "ostrich with its head in the sand" because she was not spending every waking moment trying to cure Jonathan's tumor. Annette, however, refused to accept the inevitability of death for Jonathan. She trusted their neurosurgeon and believed that Dan was over-reacting in his growing lack of confidence in the doctor. She had the hope that Jonathan's tumor would not grow, but if it did, that he would just have surgery again. She refused to believe the neurosurgeon's prognosis of three to five years. In the meantime she tried to keep family life going on as normally as possible. She continued her redecorating projects, continued her work schedule, continued her involvement with the nursery school and with the play group. She and Dan had come home from work one day to discover that Debbie, their baby-sitter, had taught Jonathan how to ride his two-wheel bike without training wheels! He was just over four years old, and already he could ride a bike! Annette felt affirmation that Jonathan was fine . . . *Look, world! Our son has a brain tumor, but he's fine . . . He can ride a bike!*

Yet, daily, Jonathan's "death sentence" would surface to her consciousness; she still felt as if she were in a nightmare from which she couldn't wake up. She wanted to share with Dan the emotions of sadness and fear that regularly overcame her, but he didn't want to discuss emotions; he wanted to discuss the medical articles he had read that day. She felt that Dan was totally obsessed with his phone calls to doctors and the hope of finding one who could help Jonathan.

A breakthrough for Dan in his battle against the tumor came when a co-worker gave him a copy of a survey from *Town and Country* magazine. The survey listed different medical specialties and some of the facilities and doctors throughout the country who dealt in these specialties. Dan finally felt as though he had leaped a major hurdle; he now had additional sources from which to begin an extensive networking telephone campaign. He began going in early to work and spending his lunch hours on the WATS line. He called every doctor and facility on the list, as well as those cited in the various articles and medical books he had been studying. He was often able to get straight through to the doctor by introducing himself as "Dr. Tomal," which he could legitimately do since he had a Ph.D. He would describe Jonathan's tumor in detail, the previous resection of part of the tumor, and request a suggested course of treatment. Some doctors would give their recommendation over the phone; other doctors would request that he mail Jonathan's CAT scans and pathology report before they would give an opinion. Upon learning that the nationally renowned clinic had already given their opinion, many doctors would respond with puzzlement, "Why are you calling me? You've already consulted _____ "—with the implication that this clinic *is* the "Mecca" and its opinion should be taken as the final answer. Dan would always finish a conversation by asking for names of other doctors who also dealt with children's brain tumors.

Throughout the next month Dan obtained more and more names of doctors and spent hours and hours talking to them, getting copies of Jonathan's CAT scans and pathology report, mailing them off to the doctors who wanted them, eagerly awaiting the daily mail, hoping for letters from doctors who were providing their opinions. He became more adept at asking the "right" questions, such as "How many astrocytoma tumors in the cerebellum on the brain stem in four-year-old children do you treat in a year?" Treatment recommendations ranged from radiation (one from an institution that he later found out had been awarded a grant to conduct a study on radiation of brain tumors), to chemotherapy, to doing nothing, to attempting more resection. He became increasingly upset at the seemingly self-serving interests portrayed by some of the doctors, especially when they asked him about health-insurance coverage before they would discuss Jonathan's case.

Even though Annette personally felt that Dan was too obsessed with Jonathan's tumor and his fight to find a cure, which she felt was impossible, she cooperated and typed up pages and pages of notes from each of his phone conversations with doctors and hospitals. Dan still was angry with

Annette and his inability to get her to discuss the different doctors' opinions. He just could not get through to her that time was limited for Jonathan and that it was up to *them* to save their son. He needed someone to help him think through and process all the contradictory information that he was getting from all the various doctors. What should their next step be?

Finally, Annette realized the truth of what Dan had been trying to drum into her . . . that it was truly up to *them*, as parents, to save their little boy's life. What turned her thinking around? Jonathan's headaches suddenly became much more frequent and severe. Seeing her little boy lying on the couch in pain, sometimes hour after hour, tore into her heart. She watched with utter sadness as his little friends played outside in the April sunshine, and she wished fervently that Jonathan could be out there with them.

What especially put Annette together with Dan in his war against the tumor was their next visit to their neurosurgeon. Told of the frequency and severity of Jonathan's headaches, his only suggestion was to put him on Decadron, a steroid. He also said that more surgery would be indicated when Jonathan got "bad." Dan and Annette were furious. How "bad" did Jonathan have to get? He was already practically a vegetable on the couch for much of the day. How much worse did he have to get? And would it be too late? The neurosurgeon still did not want to do more surgery and still would not send them elsewhere for help. It finally dawned on Annette that this doctor truly did *not* know very much about Jonathan's brain tumor, that many of the doctors Dan had been talking to seemed to have much more forceful opinions and recommendations. What long-term good would being on Decadron do, besides dulling the pain? The tumor was still there . . . and, more important, would finally cause Jonathan's symptoms to be more severe and pronounced.

*What do you do when you no longer trust your doctor?* wondered Annette as she stared out the window at the neighborhood children. Their only doctor, "Dr. I-Don't-Know" was slowly leading them to the cemetery. The realization that they were truly on their own sank into Annette's heart like an iron weight. After all, no doctor had ever called *them* with a solution; and certainly some savior wasn't about to appear on their doorstep one day and take charge of their problem.

She recalled how Dan, during visit after visit, would show their neurosurgeon his lists of doctors and facilities and how the doctor would dismiss the lists as though he felt that Dan was wasting his time talking to other doctors. Was their doctor being selfish and egocentric by refusing to give up one of his patients to the care of a doctor who would perhaps be more qualified? Another point about their doctor that had been bothering them was that whenever he prescribed a new medication for Jonathan—a sedative for a CAT scan or the Decadron—the doctor would spend such a long time studying the PDR (the book used by medical personnel that lists every drug, recommended dosages, and potential side effects), suggesting that perhaps he didn't deal very often with children with the same medical problem and symptoms that Jonathan exhibited. Annette turned from the window and looked at her once energetic, now lethargic, swollen son, and realized that time was, truly, running out . . . The clock was ticking.

One day soon afterward, as Annette was going through the mail, reading over responses from doctors regarding treatments for Jonathan, she came across a worn copy of a two-year-old *Reader's Digest* article. She read the title, something about "Aaron Alligator," and put the article in the pile of magazines and articles that Dan was attempting to plow through in his attempts to find any new procedures or technology being done that might be helpful for Jonathan. The next day, Annette's mother mailed a newspaper clipping about a New York doctor, Fred Epstein, who operated on children's brain tumors. The name *Dr. Epstein,*rang a bell for Annette; she remembered that he was the doctor written about in the *Reader's Digest* article about "Aaron Alligator" that had arrived the day before. Dr. Epstein was a pediatric neurosurgeon from New York University Medical Center and had saved the life of a little boy from Denver who had the same type of tumor as Jonathan's but along the entire spinal cord. That evening, she showed both the *Reader's Digest* article and the newspaper clipping to Dan. "What do you think, Dan? Should you call this doctor?" "Well," Dan hesitated, "I wonder if those kinds of articles are just hyped to attract readers, but I'll call him tomorrow anyway."

Dan called Dr. Epstein, who insisted over the phone, without even seeing Jonathan's CAT scans, that he would be able to completely resect his tumor even with part of it on the brain stem. Dan found that hard to believe but went ahead and sent Jonathan's CAT scans and pathology report to Dr. Epstein. Days later, Dr. Epstein called Annette personally one evening while Dan was away on a business trip and told her, "I do hundreds of these cases a year . . . hundreds. I *know* I can remove all of Jonathan's tumor." His closing remark was, "Don't be one of the parents who put off surgery and find that they waited too long." Annette was excited and could not wait to talk with Dan when he called later that evening. Dr. Epstein sounded too good to be true! Could he just be a great salesman? Dan and Annette were extremely impressed with Dr. Epstein's confidence but felt that he was being overly optimistic and that no one could so strongly state that a surgery would be near one hundred percent successful. They were skeptical but did remember that their neurosurgeon had told them that he did only a couple of such surgeries a year, and Dr. Epstein did *hundreds*. They prayed to God for guidance. That week, tentative smiles began emerging. Hope had been given to them.

Dan continued to call his list of doctors, which, at this point, was actually getting smaller because Dan would now more quickly strike off the names of obviously inadequate doctors and facilities, asking their opinions of different doctors whose names seemed to keep coming up. He now added Dr. Epstein's name to that list. Most doctors responded with comments like "He certainly is a confident guy" or "He does seem to be an excellent doctor," but although many doctors spoke well of Dr. Epstein's abilities, still no strong consensus of opinion was apparent. Annette continued to compile typewritten notes of Dan's phone conversations, including doctors' assessments of other doctors. What Dan found most interesting was the fact that doctors to whom Dan had talked earlier who had never mentioned Dr. Epstein's name or any other pediatric neurosurgeon were *now* candidly proffering their opinion of Dr. Epstein and even saying that "Epstein is probably one of the top physicians for this type of problem." Dan became very frustrated. He wanted to say to the doctors: "Why didn't *you* tell me about Epstein when I called you a month ago? Why did I have to be the one to come up with his name?"

It was now nearing the end of April, and Jonathan's headaches were getting more severe and frequent—so much so that his dose of Decadron was slowly being increased. Dan and Annette were also becoming aware of rumors spreading through their town that Jonathan's tumor was highly malignant and that Jonathan had only months to live.

On their next visit to their neurosurgeon for Jonathan's scheduled CAT scan, he told them that the tumor was still not growing and that he still did not recommend surgery but would try again if they really wanted him to. Dan told the doctor that they were going elsewhere and asked whom he would recommend from their list of doctors. The doctor sidestepped the issue and began talking about his recent trip to Atlanta, reiterating his desire that Jonathan stay under his care. Finally, Dan looked at the doctor and point-blank told him, "We're leaving. Whom should we go to?" The doctor finally studied the list. He said that Dr. Epstein was overly confident and was probably just a "good salesman." He recommended that if they insisted on taking Jonathan elsewhere, he should be taken to the children's hospital either in Ohio or in Michigan. Because a leading pediatric neurosurgeon at Michigan had already consistently come up in Dan's conversations with doctors, they decided to go there. Dan told the doctor, "We're going to Michigan." That was the last time they saw or talked with that doctor who had dangled their son's fate in his hands for so many months. Was it too late?

By the day of the appointment in Michigan the following week, Jonathan's headaches were getting still more lengthy and severe, even with the increased Decadron. He still had many good periods throughout any given day, when he would play with his friends. He still went to nursery school, where they had installed a cot for his use when he had a headache. Looking at Jonathan, anyone could tell that there was obviously something wrong with him. His face was especially puffed and swollen, as was the rest of his body, from taking so much Decadron.

On their way to the appointment, Dan and Annette felt desperate. Had they waited too long? They continued to pray for guidance. Would this doctor be able to help

Jonathan? Before they were scheduled to see the doctor, they were told to bring Jonathan to the MRI Center for an MRI of the brain. The Magnetic Resonance Imaging unit was at that time very new technology and could delineate masses inside the body better than X-ray or CAT scans could. They told the technician that since Jonathan never needed sedation anymore for CAT scans, he would not need a sedative for the MRI. How wrong they were. Jonathan was forced to lie absolutely still for almost an hour in the long, extremely narrow tube in which he was totally encased—a circumstance in which even adults usually need sedation because of the extreme claustrophobia it engenders. A humorous ending to the MRI session was that Jonathan had been allowed to wear his Voltron belt into the MRI machine; the belt buckle was totally demagnetized when Jonathan came out of the tube.

Back in the waiting room, feeling tense and anxious as they waited for their turn to see the doctor, they were at last shepherded into a small treatment room. As they talked with the nurse and learned that this neurosurgeon is a Christian, Dan and Annette felt peace that they had made the right decision in coming to this doctor. The neurosurgeon walked in and greeted Dan and Annette. She had Jonathan's MRI scans with her and explained that indeed the tumor was in a dangerous spot; it was definitely growing on the brain stem. Before she had the opportunity even to examine Jonathan, Dan handed her the list of doctors that had been narrowed down to just a few. She took the list and with just a quick glance looked up at Dan and stated, almost sternly, "You've talked to Dr. Epstein! He is probably the best in the country. You don't need me or anyone else—go to him!" The visit had ended almost as quickly as it had begun. It was time to go home and pack their bags for New York.

# 5

# New York—God's Triumph

*On the hour-long trip* back to their home, there was an air of excitement in the car. Dan and Annette both finally felt as though a tremendous burden had been lifted off their shoulders. A decision had been made. They had finally selected a pediatric neurosurgeon, after countless phone calls and after weeks of work, frustration, and pain. Their hearts kept racing, hoping that they had not waited too long. They kept thinking of Jonathan's MRI scan that showed that the tumor had grown onto the brain stem. Hopefully, Dr. Epstein would be able to save their son! All that mattered was getting Jonathan to New York as quickly as possible.

Halfway home, they stopped at Annette's college. Annette jumped out of the car and bounded into the building and into the administration office and announced to John and Carolyn, her bosses, "We're going to New York!" They looked shocked but hugged Annette tightly and said, "We will all be praying for you and Jonathan."

Once home, Dan and Annette were determined to give Jonathan a fun-filled afternoon. The neurosurgeon had increased Jonathan's dosage of Decadron, so he was feeling no pain at the moment. For late April, the weather was unseasonably warm (in the low 80s), so they got out all the "water" toys—the Slip & Slide, the sprinkler, the wading pool—and invited all the neighborhood kids over. Annette took picture after picture, capturing Jonathan laughing and playing . . . ever conscious that no one knew what Jonathan would be like after this next surgery.

That evening after the children were in bed, Annette went through the bills—writing checks for payments that would need to be made through the next month (they had no idea how long they would need to be in New York). She called her church's women's group so that a prayer for them and Jonathan could make its way through the prayer chain. She packed their clothes—very few for Jonathan but both winter and summer clothes for Stephanie and Dan and herself—who knew what the weather would be like in New York for the next month or so?

Dan called Dr. Epstein's office and was told to check Jonathan in on Sunday evening, May 4, just days away. Dan began making arrangements with his office. Marathon Oil Company, his employer, was extremely generous. The company made all the flight and travel arrangements and let them use a company car to drive to the airport. They also gave them the use of their company-leased suite at the Hotel Dorset on 53rd and Fifth. During their entire three-week stay in New York, Dan and Annette were able to use the suite every night except one.

The family flew out on Saturday, May 3, almost five months to the day that they'd been told the devastating news that Jonathan had a brain tumor. Anxiety set in. *Are we doing the right thing? . . . Is it too late for Jonathan? . . . But we have no choice . . . We hope Dr. Epstein truly is the best . . . Have we done all we can?* They arrived in New York in mid-afternoon and were immediately caught up in the city's frenetic pace. Their hotel was just five blocks away from Central Park and was a lovely, stately building. Their suite even had a balcony from which they could overlook nearby buildings. Annette and Dan were fascinated by all the adjacent rooftop gardens and how people were determined to make themselves a home, even in this vast city.

On Sunday morning, Dan and Annette and the children enjoyed some of the splendid sights of the city, including a trip to Battery Park. After taking the subway back up to midtown, they enjoyed a leisurely walk before returning to the hotel. As they walked down the Avenue of the Americas, they passed the NBC Building and Radio City Music Hall. Dan, who had been relaxed and totally enjoying the day of sightseeing, suddenly tensed and felt anxious. "What are we doing casually walking around New York? We have to go check Jonathan into the hospital." Even though Annette felt that they still had plenty of time, since it was only 4:00 P.M., Dan's tension had invaded their relaxing afternoon. The fun time had ended. Reality had once again set in. They quickly returned to the hotel, packed Jonathan's and Annette's bags, grabbed sandwiches from a street vendor, hailed a taxi, and were at NYU Medical Center promptly at 6:00 o'clock.

The hospital was on First Avenue and next to the East River. The lobby inside was vast, and they waited for over an hour for their turn to check in. As they stepped out of the elevator onto the pediatric floor, both Dan and Annette were stopped dead in their tracks at the shocking sight of the other children . . . children with bald heads and long surgical scars, children with huge bandages down the backs of their heads or the sides of their heads or around their heads, children with deformed faces, children who were lively and energetic, children who were listless, children who were like large, overgrown toddlers. . . . All kinds of medical problems were represented here. Dan felt as though he were entering a "war zone," but he just looked at Annette and said, "This is the right place!" Jonathan fit right in—it was totally unlike the first hospital where most of the other

children were beset by problems no more serious than
hernias and tonsillectomies.

After Dan and Stephanie left, Annette and Jonathan
settled into their room. Annette was given a cot. Their
roommate for the evening was a six-year-old boy with a
problem that was minor in comparison to most of the cases
on the floor. The mother was a friendly, vivacious native
New Yorker who lived just several blocks away and invited
Annette to stop by some afternoon while in New York.
Soon two medical students arrived to take Annette and
Jonathan to a treatment room. Jonathan's medical history
was taken, and his blood was drawn. He was taken
downstairs for a CAT scan—deep down into the caverns of
the immense hospital. Annette was told that surgery would
definitely not be the next day . . . perhaps the day after . . .
perhaps not for several days; Dr. Epstein was extremely busy
these days.

The next day was long but in a strange way, uplifting.
The camaraderie among the other parents was therapeutic,
as they had finally found other people with whom they had
something in common. These parents could share their fear,
their concern, their feelings of helplessness, their emotional
pain and suffering, their hopes that Dr. Epstein would be
able to help their child. Strangely, as Dan and Annette
listened to the other parents' tragic experiences, they
actually felt "relief" that Jonathan "only" had a brain tumor.
Eventually, they realized that most of the parents felt this
way—that no matter how serious the medical problem of
their own child, each parent felt unable to cope with
anything else.

Dan and Annette marveled at how God helps parents
cope; when they are around other children with serious
problems, parents actually become *thankful*—and yet, *all*
the parents seem to feel that other families' problems are

worse than their own. In other words, they realize that God gives a person strength to cope with a particular problem and that he helps a person to perceive other people's problems to be worse. Self-pity, therefore, disappears, and prayers of thanksgiving take its place.

Stephanie was now thirteen months old and had learned to walk just a few weeks earlier. She had a great time toddling around the waiting room, pretending to get on the elevator, and greeting people as they arrived on the pediatric floor. She insisted on drinking her bottle on another parent's lap. Jonathan had a great time playing the computer games in the toy room.

Finally, at the end of the day, Dr. Epstein and his associate came to see them and announced that surgery would be the next morning. The fear and anxiety returned as he explained the possible risks and complications. Dr. Epstein explained that with the tumor on the brain stem, the surgery was risky and would be much more difficult than the first surgery and that recovery would be much longer and harder. He was confident, however, and anticipated that a more serious type and grade of tumor would be unlikely.

Annette called her mother, who had offered to fly to New York from Indiana to care for Stephanie on the day of the surgery and the following day. She would fly out the next morning. That was a long evening for Dan in the hotel room with Stephanie and for Annette in the hospital room with Jonathan. Jonathan's roommate for the night was a twenty-year-old, severely brain-damaged boy who screamed and moaned all night long. Luckily, at least Jonathan was finally able to sleep, but he woke up at 6:00 A.M.—starving. Dan and Annette felt sorry for the hungry little boy as they tried to distract him with toys and activities all through the long hours of the morning. His grandma's arrival was a highlight of the morning. Finally, at 1:00 P.M., an orderly came to take Jonathan to surgery.

Annette went with Jonathan down the hallway and down the elevator, where she kissed him good-bye. As she watched him being wheeled on a hospital bed down the long corridor toward the huge doors of the surgical operating rooms, she broke down and turned to the wall, rested her forehead on it, and sobbed and sobbed. A nurse came up to her and put her arm around Annette's shoulders. "He'll be okay. He's in good hands," she said.

Annette's mom and Stephanie spent the entire afternoon in the toy room. Dan and Annette felt a strong need to get out of the hospital setting, where their fears were uppermost in their minds. Would Jonathan be okay? Would he end up paralyzed? Would the brain tumor be too far into the brain stem? Would Dr. Epstein be able to get the whole tumor out? For a few short hours, they were able to put those fears out of their minds as they walked the streets of New York— over to Fifth Avenue, where they window-shopped—and finally to FAO Schwartz near Central Park, where they bought Jonathan lots of He-Man toys.

All of a sudden they both wanted to be back in the hospital. What if something had gone wrong? No one knew where they were. They frantically flagged down a taxi to take them back to the hospital. They dashed up to the pediatric floor and into the toy room where Stephanie and her grandma were busy dressing dolls. One look at Annette's mom's calm face let them know that nothing had happened and that surgery was still going on.

Finally, at 7:00 P.M., Dr. Epstein walked into the toy room. "Everything's fine," he announced. "We got it all." Dan grabbed Annette and hugged her tightly. He grabbed his mother-in-law and hugged her tightly. He looked at Dr.

Epstein with tears in his eyes and said, "Praise God! Thank you! Thank you so much!"

Stephanie left with her grandmother to go to the Ronald McDonald House, where they would spend the next two nights. Dan and Annette waited anxiously for several more hours for Jonathan to be brought back to the floor. Finally, at 1:00 A.M.—twelve hours after Jonathan had been wheeled into surgery—he was back on the pediatric floor and being wheeled into the ICU. Dan and Annette's hearts stuck in their throats upon seeing all the tubes and bandages, and Jonathan lying so still. Dan sat next to Jonathan in ICU the rest of the night while Annette slept on the floor of the toy room. Finally, at 6:00 A.M., Jonathan awoke. Dan jumped up and looked down at him. The boy looked horrible—his eyes were spinning, he couldn't focus, he couldn't talk, and he had tubes and monitors hooked up to him. When Dan and Annette looked at the other children in ICU, they were scared. They saw the little boy next to Jonathan die that afternoon; they saw a little baby completely wrapped in bandages, with nurses constantly hovering over him; they saw parents weeping in agony.

Annette spent that night with her mother and Stephanie at Ronald McDonald House. Getting into a taxi, she told the driver her destination and the address. During the drive, she could not stop thinking about Jonathan—so helpless, those eyes spinning around, still not talking. How long would it be before they would know if he was okay? As the driver approached the house, he realized that he was going down the street in the wrong direction and brusquely asked Annette why she had not told him which way he should be going. She said, "That's okay; I can cross the street; you don't have to turn around." The driver swung the car in a screeching U-turn and snapped, "You should have told me which side I was supposed to be on." Annette suddenly burst into tears. "What did I do?" asked the driver in bewilderment and embarrassment as Annette stood on the sidewalk with tears running down her face. Two pedestrians stopped to ask Annette if she was okay. "I didn't do anything!" protested the driver. "Just leave me alone," sobbed Annette. "My little boy has a brain tumor." The pressure had just been too much. She grabbed her suitcase and rushed into the Ronald McDonald House.

As she tried to compose herself in the little waiting room, she noticed a large, gorgeous bouquet of spring flowers with a card reading, "Dan and Annette Tomal." Opening the card, she felt tears come again to her eyes, this time tears of joy and appreciation: The Women's Circle in their church had sent the flowers. Lying next to the flowers was a wrapped package addressed to Jonathan; inside was an electronic Nintendo pocket game, also from the Women's Circle. There was also a picture of all the children from Jonathan's Sunday school class holding a big sign reading, "We miss you, Jonathan. Get well soon." What thoughtful friends they had back home.

Stephanie had adjusted very well to staying with her grandma and slept in a playpen in their room. The Ronald McDonald House was big, having several floors with many bedrooms. Many families stayed there at any given time. There was a kitchen and a huge living room that all the families shared. Some families were there from Europe and South America and had been there for weeks; almost all their children had some form of cancer and were being treated at any of the New York hospitals. Listening to the other parents' problems made Annette sad. Would she be like this in a few weeks, still in New York, talking with other parents about her son's progress, so out-of-touch with the outside world, totally wrapped up in the day-to-day care of her child?

The next day was a gorgeous, sunny May day with temperatures in the 70s. Annette, her mom, and Stephanie enjoyed the long walk back to the hospital, stopping in one of the many coffee shops along the way for a leisurely breakfast. Stephanie was so cute, standing up on her seat and "talking" to the other patrons. They walked down 34th Street, the section of the city with the clothing warehouses, and watched with fascination the racks of clothes being wheeled from delivery trucks into cramped doorways.

Once back at the hospital, they all went up to the pediatric floor. What a switch—going from the gorgeous sunshine and the throngs of people and the bustle of activity into the quiet and the medicinal smell of the hospital containing the children with bald heads from chemotherapy treatment and the children with scars and bandages. *Let us out, dear God; do we have to be here?*

Annette's mom left to fly back home. Now Dan, Annette, and Stephanie settled into what would become their routine for the remainder of their three-week stay at NYU Medical Center. Jonathan remained in ICU for two days before being moved to a room on the pediatric floor. He had four more roommates during the rest of his hospital stay. One was a tiny baby born with a horribly deformed face, who would need many surgeries during the next few years before he would look even somewhat normal. Another child was a toddler with Down's Syndrome, who had pneumonia. The next roommate was a listless, lethargic baby with spina bifida, who lay in her crib all day; her parents only visited for about a half hour every evening. The final roommate was a gorgeous toddler who had had a calcium mass successfully removed from his brain.

Dan and Annette took twenty-four hour shifts with Jonathan, sleeping in a cot next to his bed while the other went every evening to the hotel with Stephanie. Stephanie learned to hail taxis, raising her arm out as taxis went racing by. Luckily, every single day of the entire three weeks was sunny and in the 70s. They both enjoyed their twice-daily walks to the hospital from the hotel, with Stephanie in her stroller. The slow walk to the hospital was a necessary mental and emotional break for them before facing the rest of the day in the hospital. Jonathan was recovering so slowly. The spinal fluid continually bulged out the back of his head where a piece of his skull had been taken out so that the surgery could be done. To drain the excess spinal fluid, one of Dr. Epstein's staff came in daily to aspirate the excess fluid with a long needle. The aspiration was very painful for Jonathan; the drastic change in the amount of fluid in his head caused severe, sudden head pain. Soon, the mere sight of that staff member walking into the room caused Jonathan to burst out screaming. He had regular blood tests, some necessitating several attempts and needle pricks before blood was drawn. He had to be spoon-fed. He was on massive doses of steroids because of the pain and swelling.

The only time that Jonathan smiled was when little Stephanie walked into the room. She was always cheerful and outgoing. One of the other mothers called her "Miss Stephanie." In this hospital, though, Jonathan did not need to wear a hat to cover his bandage; he was just "one of the crowd" here. Eventually Jonathan felt well enough to be carried down to the toy room, where Stephanie would pull him around in a tiny wagon. Jonathan could not crawl or walk, had no coordination, and the recovery period still brought periods of renewed fear. More than one child had died during his or her stay at the hospital. One of the mothers continuously filled their heads with horror stories of the possibility of permanent brain and nerve damage, but Dan and Annette dismissed her comments, knowing that Jonathan was improving. At one point, the staff was concerned that Jonathan might be developing meningitis. Another time, they became concerned about his liver and kidneys, so Jonathan had to have another CAT scan.

Finally the day came when Jonathan had his first post-operative CAT scan of his brain. Afterward, Dan and Annette were asked to report to Dr. Epstein's office to look at the CAT scan. Dr. Epstein's associate pinned up the CAT scan on the view box and showed them the spot where the tumor had been. The CAT scan showed a large, black circle. "Is that where the tumor was?" asked Annette. "You mean, that whole time in Ohio, that tiny, black spot on the CAT scan was not just the remainder of the tumor but actually was only what had been taken out in the first surgery?" Seeing that large, black hole where the tumor had been was a moment of triumph. They finally truly believed Dr. Epstein. When he had said, "We got it all" following the surgery, he had been right. They were finally convinced that the tumor had been excised.

Even after seeing the CAT scan with the convincing big black hole and even seeing Jonathan slowly getting more alert and regaining his hand-eye coordination, Dan still would regularly sneak down to the medical library to read and copy everything he could about brain tumors. It was hard for him to get out of that habit that he had been programmed into for the last few months. One evening he asked Dr. Epstein a very technical question about grading characteristics of an astrocytoma relative to prognosis. Dr. Epstein looked at him and said, "You are getting too smart. You don't need to keep studying. Your son is going to be fine. Let's get Jonathan well so that you can all go home." Dan was startled. He finally realized that his obsession with finding the right doctor had paid off, and he felt a great burden lifted from his shoulders.

From then on, Dan made it his goal to get Jonathan

walking again. He spent increasing amounts of time every day working with Jonathan in the hallway, holding on to him, encouraging him, pushing him to keep walking a few more steps, eventually seeing Jonathan take a step on his own and then two steps, until finally he could make a wobbly path of his own from his room down to the toy room.

The days began to stretch into weeks as Jonathan totally occupied Dan and Annette's minds and emotions. They longed to be home. A break for them came when one of the parents volunteered to watch Stephanie while they went to the cafeteria for a cup of coffee. This was the first time they had been alone together since arriving in New York. Going down in the elevator, they realized how abnormal the whole lifestyle at the hospital was. They just wanted to be home, back in the routine of work and raising kids. As they finished their coffee and were heading back up in the elevator, they also realized that such is life—much like the elevator—with all its ups and downs, trials and tribulations, happiness and sadness—in which the ups and downs may vary from person to person, but from which no one can escape.

The days continued to be long and hard, attending to Jonathan's every need, changing shifts daily. After two weeks of the intense schedule, a welcome call came to Dan. It was from a close co-worker, Rick, who would be coming to New York on business and would have to use their suite for the night. Rick invited Dan and Stephanie to stay with him. Putting Stephanie to sleep early that evening, the two of them crawled out the window onto the balcony. Like two college kids, they spent the evening viewing the big city's night life with all the noise, busy streets, and brightly lit windows. Rick was able to get Dan's mind off Jonathan that evening, a night that Dan would always appreciate as a much-needed emotional and mental break.

Jonathan began spending time with an occupational

therapist in his room and in the toy room. She was amazed at his superior eye-hand coordination and his ability to do jigsaw puzzles; she said that he was above average for even "normal" four-year-olds, so she discontinued the occupational therapy. Jonathan and Stephanie began playing together more frequently in the toy room; Stephanie continued to push Jonathan around the room in the little wooden wagon because he still was unable to walk well.

Finally, Dr. Epstein started talking about the Tomals' returning to Ohio. Unfortunately, Jonathan developed a fever, and the fear again was that Jonathan was developing meningitis. After several days, however, the morning came when the nurse announced that Jonathan was afebrile (no fever) and Dr. Epstein said that they could fly back home! It was Saturday, May 24: They had been in New York exactly three weeks.

# Back Home—
# God's Final Victory

*In the taxi, suitcases in the trunk,* Dan and Annette gazed out the windows for one long last look at New York—their home for the last three weeks. They both felt an odd attachment to the city and its never ending hustle-bustle of activity. As they sped through the Lincoln Tunnel and eventually were out of Manhattan heading for Newark Airport, they both felt as though they were experiencing culture shock; they could actually see into the distance. There were wide-open spaces; there were fields. New York was truly a world of its own, and they finally realized how people could become so engrossed in the life of that tiny island that the rest of the United States seemed almost like a foreign country.

On their way back home from the airport in Detroit, they stopped at Toys R Us and let Jonathan pick out several toys—whatever he wanted. He picked out games and He-Man vehicles. Finally, they pulled into their driveway. It was a beautiful spring day, and all the neighborhood children came running over to their car. "Jonathan! Jonathan!" they screamed. Their cries of joy changed to shock as they watched Dan get out of the car, open the back door, and carry Jonathan out. "Can't he walk?" one boy asked. "He'll walk again, don't worry," Annette responded. "He's still getting better from the surgery." A couple of the children came into the house with them and played one of the new games with Jonathan. Very soon, however, Jonathan wanted to lie down; he was tired and had a headache. As Dan carried the suitcases upstairs, his eyes caught a glimpse of the upstairs study. He stopped for a moment as he stared at the stately rolltop desk sitting there, and he thought, *There is no "life guarantee" in the drawer. Life is just a thread of string that could be snipped at any time.* The moment made him realize the mortality of man, the preciousness of life, and the vulnerability that we all have.

Jonathan was far from being recovered. He still had an incision of approximately eight inches in diameter where his skull had literally been drilled and sawed open. This area at the back of his head was very soft, much like a newborn baby's soft spot but with a golf ball-size sac of spinal fluid bulging the flesh outward. Dr. Epstein had warned them that Jonathan would probably need a shunt to control this collection of fluid and the potential hydrocephalus.

Two days later, on Memorial Day, Jonathan developed such an extremely severe headache that Dan and Annette called their pediatrician and met her at the emergency room. She was quite frank with them and told them that she felt "out of her league" with this problem and that they really needed to call someone more qualified. They called the pediatric neurosurgeon in Michigan, the doctor who had sent them to Dr. Epstein in the first place. She told them not to worry but to call if Jonathan got worse.

The next day, Dan returned to work, and Annette stayed home with Jonathan and Stephanie. She realized that her daily routine would not return to normal for a long time. To distract Jonathan from his pain, she found herself reading to him, playing tapes to him, playing games with him—all the while trying to keep her eye on Stephanie. At one point, she looked out in the backyard and saw Stephanie at the top of the slide of the swingset. She was only fourteen months old, and Annette ran out to make sure that she was okay. Stephanie smiled and laughed as Annette rushed up, and Annette realized that she was fine. By the time she came back into the family room, Jonathan was crying for her to read him another book.

By the middle of the afternoon, however, Annette realized that something was very wrong. Jonathan was getting extremely lethargic, his eyes looked glazed, and most important, she noticed that fluid was starting to seep out of the wound in the back of his head. With growing concern, she called Dan for the second time at his office, trying to impress upon him Jonathan's worsening condition, insisting that he call the pediatric neurosurgeon in Michigan. The neurosurgeon told Dan to get Jonathan to the Michigan hospital immediately. The spinal fluid was building up to an excessive level in Jonathan's brain, and the doctor feared that infection would set in due to the leakage.

Again, Annette went into action. She called their neighbor Debbie to see if she would watch Stephanie again for who-knew-how-long. She called the church's prayer chain and relayed the news that they were taking Jonathan back to the hospital. She began packing clothes for herself and Jonathan as well as books and toys. The minister called and asked if he could come over. Annette said, "No, thank you. I really appreciate your offer, but I have to pack so that we can leave as soon as Dan gets home." The minister called Dan, who was still at work, and said that he was concerned that Annette did not want him over. Dan thanked him for his concern but told him that she probably just wanted to get the packing done because they did have to get Jonathan to the hospital immediately. As she packed, Annette forced her mind to concentrate even though it was whirling around like a dervish. What now? Would they get Jonathan there on time? Panic again set in.

As soon as Dan got home, they took off—Dan driving and Annette in the back seat, cradling Jonathan's head. Dan drove fast, lights flashing, horn honking. Most cars immediately got out of their way; sometimes a driver would stubbornly remain in their lane and refuse to pull over. Finally, ninety miles later, they arrived at the Michigan hospital.

They rushed into the emergency room, Dan carrying Jonathan, who by now was limp and in continuous pain. The staff directed them to the proper treatment room where one of the neurosurgeon's residents was already waiting for them. He informed Dan and Annette that he would be inserting a huge needle into Jonathan's spinal column to begin withdrawing spinal fluid and that it would be extremely painful for Jonathan. He suggested that they might not want to stay and watch. "Of course, we'll stay," they responded. It was agony for both of them as they watched the doctor inject a long needle into Jonathan's spine and watch as Jonathan screamed in pain. Annette stroked Jonathan's arms and back, but tears welled in her eyes. How much more would her poor little boy have to take?

The next week was absolute misery for Jonathan. For Annette, this week was the absolute worst yet. Jonathan suffered terrible, horrible pain that week. The doctor decided to relieve the spinal fluid buildup in Jonathan's brain by inserting a tube into Jonathan's spinal column; attached to the outside of the tube was a valve and a bag to collect the excess fluid. Jonathan had to lie absolutely, completely immobile for twenty-four hours a day for seven days as the fluid drained out of his skull, down the tube, and into its receptacle bag. Every time he moved, excruciating pain and agony shot through Jonathan because of the change in the spinal fluid pressure. Regularly, the doctor came in to adjust the valve to cause the fluid to drain either more slowly or more quickly. Each time, the adjustment caused Jonathan tremendous pain as the fluid pressure changed so quickly. Within a couple of days, Jonathan would stiffen and cringe every time he heard footsteps behind him, fearing that it was the doctor coming to adjust the valve again. Annette read him book after book and played him tape after tape—trying desperately to keep his mind off his immobility and pain. She often wondered if she and Dan were being selfish—did they have the right to put their little boy through so much agony just so they could have their son alive? *Thank God that Jonathan never, ever asked his parents why he was going through such suffering. Thank God that Jonathan was so young and still looked at his parents with blind, adoring faith.* Years later, Darla (Annette's good friend from work) recalled that when she had visited Jonathan in the hospital that week, she cried and cried once she was back in her car. She had been convinced that Jonathan was not going to live; he looked so very much worse than he had before going to New York.

Annette stayed in the hospital that long week caring for Jonathan; Dan stayed home, working during the day and caring for Stephanie in the evening. Finally, at the end of the week, the neurosurgeon realized that this temporary measure was not helping Jonathan. She decided to surgically implant a shunt that ran down his spinal column and around to his stomach for drainage. The surgery went well. Two nights later, however, as the neurosurgeon was checking the surgical site of the valve, the wound suddenly broke and spinal fluid began gushing straight up into the air. Jonathan was rushed into emergency surgery and eventually came back in the middle of the night from the recovery room.

The shunt surgery was successful; Jonathan finally began to start feeling better. Soon Annette began pushing him around the hospital in his wheelchair, even venturing onto the roof of the building, where there was a small playground. They began spending more and more time in the toy room. Jonathan's headaches were minimal. The only remaining, painful part of the hospitalization was Jonathan's daily blood tests. The technicians had begun using Jonathan's foot because he was running out of unused veins; it still usually took several pokes before a blood draw was successful. Jonathan was so brave, though, that it was usually not until the third vein was tried that he would start crying.

His spirits were finally starting to pick up, and he began making friends with some of the nurses. One favorite activity was taping his He-Man characters to his bedrails so that they appeared to be standing straight up. He enjoyed the reactions of the people walking past his room as they saw his He-Man characters all lined up on his bedrails.

At this point, Annette was only going home on weekends; Dan would then stay with Jonathan in the hospital. On her first weekend home, she went to church with Stephanie but sat in the back so that she wouldn't have to face people and accept their sympathy. Even before the service ended, she found herself in tears—thinking of all the pain that Jonathan was going through and of the unknown future. She quietly left without talking to anyone. On another weekend home, she rode her bike around the block, feeling as though she were an alien in a foreign world. She felt far removed from the people weeding their gardens and mowing their lawns. As she was parking her bike in the garage, a friend from play group pulled into the driveway on her bike.

This friend had been unable to visit the hospital following Jonathan's first surgery; she just had not been able to face talking to Dan and Annette and seeing Jonathan. Seeing this friend in the driveway—the concern on her face and asking the question, "How's Jonathan doing?"—caused

Annette to break down in tears. Annette just looked at her
friend, and tears rolled down her face as she silently turned
around and walked into the house. She just could not yet
talk to people about Jonathan—knowing and feeling the pity
that they must surely feel. She felt sorry for her friend,
knowing the pain that she must have felt when her simple
question, "How's Jonathan doing?" had caused Annette to
break down in grief.

The entire ordeal had developed a strong sense of
compassion and empathy in Dan and Annette for others
going through similar hardships. They often found themselves comforting other parents as they entered the hospital
with their children. One day a couple brought their young
boy into the hospital. They were hysterical, and fear radiated
across their faces. Dan had seen that look so many times
before. He quickly approached them as he had done with so
many other parents. Eventually, he asked what was wrong
with their child. He was surprised when they responded that
their child needed to have an appendectomy. *An appendectomy; that's all?* Dan thought to himself as he proceeded to
mumble under his breath, "Don't even talk to me, you don't
even know what problems are!" He just stared at them as
they continued in their torment. The brief encounter made
him realize that people experience many varying degrees of
problems. He began to realize that there is always someone
worse off than he. He began to think that even his own
experience was nothing compared with that of many people
who live their entire life in pain, suffering, and disability,
only to find death at the end of their ordeal.

Even though Dan was feeling worn down, he knew that
Jonathan was going to recover and that the real battle—
against the tumor—had been won. He felt concerned for
Annette at this time, though, thinking of her months of close
and constant care of Jonathan, depriving herself of any

personal pleasures. Finally, after three weeks in Michigan, the doctor suggested to Annette that perhaps Jonathan was ready to go home. Annette felt panic. What if something went wrong at home? How would she know what to do? Having spent so much uninterrupted time in the hospital with Jonathan, the hospital was becoming the daily routine for Annette. One day as she sat outside in the courtyard while Jonathan napped, she watched people going in and out of the hospital—people visiting patients, employees reporting for work. Annette realized that for her the hospital *was* now her life, and she found it difficult to remember what a "normal" life of work and home was like. The doctor told Annette not to leave until she felt comfortable with caring for Jonathan, but that he really was doing fine and was ready to finish recovery at home.

So, again after a three-week stay in the hospital, Jonathan and Annette returned home. This time, recovery went much faster. Within a week Jonathan was walking. He began having friends over to play again. His headaches were infrequent and mild. He no longer looked like a "normal" little boy, however. His face and body were still swollen from all the steroids he had been on during the past months. His gait was unsteady and irregular; he often appeared clumsy as he bumped into objects as he walked. His left side was decidedly weaker and less coordinated than his right side, and his left arm tended to dangle. His eyes were slightly crossed, and he had double vision, since the pressure in his brain had affected the fourth and sixth nerves to his eyes.

Jonathan steadily improved each day. His coordination slowly became more steady and balanced. His left side slowly became stronger and more equal to his right side. He eventually began to run again. He needed one more surgery on his shunt that summer, done on an outpatient basis, before the fluid buildup in his brain seemed to be regulated normally. Still the recovery had been hard, just as Dr. Epstein had said that it would be. But Jonathan, like so many kids, seemed to bounce back quickly. Children's innocence in understanding the magnitude of their illness and their blind acceptance of their parents' decisions were so vivid to Dan and Annette as they realized the power and influence that parents have over their child's development.

Dan and Annette were still concerned for Jonathan, and though they felt confident that he was cured of the tumor, they were not totally convinced of his full recovery. They were still very protective and cautious with him, constantly worrying that he might play too hard and burst open his wound again. Even though the incision had healed well, there was no bony skull material—only a soft spot—and the fear that a sharp object might pierce the wound was a constant concern.

Then, finally, the eventful afternoon came one warm day in July. Jonathan wanted to try riding his bike again—the two-wheel bike that he had learned to ride without training wheels just weeks before going to New York. Dan was reluctant, fearing the worst. What if he should fall? Was his coordination developed enough? Could he ever ride it again? Annette pleaded with Dan to give in. "We can't protect him forever; we've got to let him try." Finally, Dan gave in as Jonathan struggled to mount his bike. It was a beautiful, sunny Sunday. Many of the neighbors were outside washing their cars, playing outdoors, or working in their yards. Dan helped Jonathan onto the bike; he slowly ran behind him and kept the bike balanced as Jonathan pedaled. The neighbors became aware of what was going on and stopped what they were doing. They stared in suspense and disbelief as they viewed the child who only months before had been destined to die. As Jonathan wobbled down the road with Dan holding on to the bike seat, he suddenly took off riding on his own! He was riding! Dan and Annette started yelling cheers, Annette started crying, the neighbors began cheering and clapping. What a momentous day! Praise God! Finally, Dan and Annette truly realized that Jonathan was totally cured and that he eventually would be totally normal. They had won! The tumor was conquered! *God had answered prayer!*

# Epilogue

The first year of Jonathan's recovery was difficult. His left side was noticeably weaker and less coordinated than his right side, although he continued to improve. He continued to suffer frequent, long headaches. He had two eye surgeries to correct strabismus and double vision. Within a couple years, then, he was eventually "back to normal." Jonathan is now twelve years old and is totally cured. His follow-up MRI scans have shown no trace of tumor, and people are surprised to learn that he had a brain tumor when he was younger. He is a typical sixth-grade boy, active in sports year-round. He squabbles with his younger sister and brother and collects baseball cards. We thank God for helping us "beat" the medical referral system and for finding Dr. Epstein in time to help Jonathan.

In our great country, people should never be told, "There is nothing that can be done for you," when, in fact, there probably *are* doctors who can help. Even after completing this book, so many questions continue to haunt us—questions that we have grappled with and discussed with each other, other people, and other health professionals—questions that are still unanswered: Why did Jonathan have to go through what he did? Why didn't the original neurosurgeon discuss with us the differences between a neurosurgeon and a pediatric neurosurgeon? Why didn't our pediatrician suggest that we go to a pediatric neurosurgeon? Why did our original neurosurgeon convince us to stay with him even after we stressed to him that we wanted the best doctor and facility in the country? Why did he never explain the CAT scans to us and instead imply that the small black hole was the remaining tumor rather than the resected tumor that it actually was? Why would a prestigious physician from a prestigious medical clinic render an opinion without ever having seen Jonathan, thereby giving validation to the first neurosurgeon's handling of the case? Why would our neurosurgeon then paraphrase that doctor's letter with his own interpretation and then relay his interpretation to us and to our own pediatrician? What were the compelling motives of the first neurosurgeon that he did not want to give up Jonathan's case? Why did he continue to shoot CAT scans on such a regular basis? Whatever the reason— ignorance, ego, greed, regionalism—it cannot justify a doctor's dangling the fate of a child's life in his hands.

Jonathan's story first appeared in *Ladies' Home Journal* in August 1991. The article led to national TV coverage: NBC "Cover to Cover," CBS "This Morning," and CBN "700 Club." Hundreds of parents from all over the country have called us after reading the article or seeing us on TV, with stories similar to ours: "Our doctor told us there's no hope for our child," or "Our doctor refuses to refer us to anyone else." We have listened to their pain, their grief, their confusion, and we have cried with them. We have tried to comfort, encourage, and direct these parents. Many of them have called us back with the good news that they were able to find the "right" doctor who saved their child.

Our country's medical referral and health-care systems should not be so difficult for people to access and utilize. People should not have to rely on their own doctor for referrals to specialists, especially when that doctor is deter- mined to hang on to the case even though better care could be provided by another physician. There needs to be a better way for people to find the right doctor or facility for a given medical problem. United States Representative Tim Roemer of Indiana is at this time working on a Congressional bill to develop a proposed "HELP" (Health Education Listing Program) network to help people nationwide find the right doctor for any medical problem through a national hotline telephone and computerized database system.

We hope that all people in this country will eventually not only be able to access the medical system to find the best doctor for their medical problems but will take charge of their own medical care.

# Part Two
# Finding the Best Doctor

# 1

# Taking Charge
# —You Can Do It!

*Would* you *know what to do* if you or your child or your spouse were faced with a serious medical problem? If your doctor were reluctant to send you elsewhere? If you keep seeing your doctor or taking your medicines and are still not improving? If you wonder whether your doctor is the best one for you? If your doctor said, "There is nothing anyone can do"?

Do not be like the thirty-year-old mother from California who is dying from cancer because her doctors told her year after year not to worry about the lump in her breast, until finally the cancer had spread throughout her body. Because this woman was reluctant to fight the medical system, she will soon die, and her three young children will grow up without a mother. Do not be like the man from Indiana who at age eighty-three was told that he was "too old" for cataract surgery and then lived to age ninety-eight. Because this man believed his doctor, he had to live out his last sixteen years in blindness, unable to enjoy his hobbies of reading and woodworking.

You cannot rely on your doctor to always give you or direct you to the best medical treatment; *you* must learn to take charge of your own medical care. *You* must learn to question your doctor and to fight the medical system when necessary. *You* have the *right* to demand the best treatment, and you must learn how to get that treatment. A practical and down-to-earth approach is presented in this part of the book to help you take charge of your medical care and find the right doctor. You will gain insight into the medical system so that you will better understand your doctor's decisions. The appendices include listings of organizations, foundations, consulting groups, medical surveys, and hotline services. Always remember—you have the *right* to access the great medical system in our country. Don't assume that your doctor will do it for you.

## The First Step

What do you do when you hear dreaded words: *cancer, chronic, tumor, inoperable, "nothing can be done"—learn to live with it—terminal?* First, let yourself acknowledge the pain, the grief, the confusion. Immerse yourself in your tears and your grief but don't let those emotions take over. Turn to prayer—*directed* prayer, not passive prayer. Passive prayer is putting your medical problem into God's hands and then sitting back and doing nothing. Directed prayer is when you specifically pray for healing and for strength, courage, patience, and direction. God works in many ways and often through people. Open yourself to God as he opens up doors for you so that you can undertake the necessary actions to resolve your medical problems. As you continue to fight your medical problems, continue to send directed prayer to God.

## Be Courageous and Manage Your Fear

One of the severest limitations to successful health care is fear. When a terrible health problem strikes, people are so afraid of the condition that it immobilizes them and puts them at the mercy of the disease and the doctor. Turn your fear around and transform it into a positive, driving force. Do not waste precious time feeling sorry for yourself and letting your fear of the disease control you. The choice is yours. You can either be courageous or be cowardly. Courage is doing the right thing despite your fear. Be assertive. Do not accept your treatment if you find yourself questioning the doctor's decisions. Whenever you feel fear and need a boost of courage, look into the eyes of your child, or your loved one. Can you afford to be a coward when your loved one is suffering?

Some people let their illness become an excuse for their laziness. They sit around complaining and feeling sorry for themselves and allow their illness to devitalize them to the point where their illness progresses to the stage of chronic pain, or death. This attitude leads to psychosomatic illness and fuels the legitimate disease. Dr. Fred Epstein once commented to a young couple whose child had a life-threatening brain tumor that, from his years of experience, parents should "take faith; those who take faith and courage seem to do better than those who don't." Take charge of your health care with faith and courage. Don't let fear overtake your life.

## Why Many People Do Not Select the Best Doctor

How would *you* select the best doctor if you have a medical problem? Most people select a doctor who is nearby, usually one recommended by their family physician, or the one with whom they can get the earliest appointment. The medical profession is more advanced than ever before, but our system for identifying and matching the right doctor with our health needs is still primitive. There are literally thousands of doctors and medical institutions, but rarely do people or the referring physician complete a thorough search for their treatment. Dr. Lawrence Horowitz, former

Director of the U.S. Senate Health Committee, states that "every day . . . patients in every city in America walk into their doctor's office seeking help. And depending on how sick they are, or how serious their illnesses are, that variation can cost them prolonged suffering, extended illness, or even their lives."[1]

You must become an educated health consumer to ensure that you receive quality health care. Dr. Arthur Levin emphasizes this point by stating, "I am amazed at how little most people know about the different places they can obtain care. . . . In most places, even rural areas, there are alternative sources of care. Consumers need not put up with doctors or hospitals who are not responsive to their needs."[2]

For several reasons, people fail to conduct a thorough search in selecting a doctor or medical facility:

1. *Knowledge*—Most people don't realize the importance of selecting the right doctor or medical facility. They do not understand that differences exist in the skills of doctors and among the quality of services of medical facilities. For example, according to one federal report, the rate of Medicare patients' dying from coronary bypass surgery in 1984 at two similar Indiana hospitals was 22.7% at one and 1.3% at the other (Federal Health Care Financing Administration). That statistic should be of vital importance to a heart patient. Other studies have shown wide disparity in physician errors, standards of health care, and patient management. This issue is further discussed in chapter 4.

2. *False-Trust-in-Doctor Syndrome*—People may not even realize that they are *supposed* to question their doctor and that they don't *have* to accept everything he or she says. People have traditionally believed that they must respect and trust their physician. This "false-trust-in-doctor" syndrome is similar to the "halo effect," in which a person sees

an individual as doing no wrong. Likewise, the patient trusts the doctor and tends not to question the doctor's judgment.

3. *Immediate Action*—Parents, especially, tend to over-react and want immediate action. Perhaps no keener pain can be felt than the pain that parents experience when their own children are suffering. Parents are, therefore, exceptionally vulnerable to the advice and opinions of any medical doctor. Even though the problem may be serious and need prompt treatment, it may not be of an emergency nature for which surgery is needed the next day. It may be advantageous for the family to take additional time before making any major decisions.

4. *Skills*—Most people have not learned the skills for initiating a search campaign, asking the right questions, and making the right decision—skills that will be presented in the following chapters.

5. *Time*—The day-to-day hectic schedules and activities can make it difficult for people to prioritize and schedule time to initiate a thorough medical search. People must learn to manage their time and reprioritize their activities during a health-care problem.

6. *Intimidation*—Many people are intimidated by doctors. They feel foolish or uncomfortable asking too many questions, especially questions about a doctor's experience or skills. Some doctors may reinforce this situation by their indifference, confusing medical jargon, or formal manner.

7. *Too Busy*—"I only saw the doctor for three minutes; how was I to ask any meaningful questions?" Some doctors don't spend much time with their patients, which makes it difficult for the patients to ask quality questions. People have a right to have their questions answered and should not settle for less. The point could be made that the best doctors are those who are probably the busiest but who still manage to give their patients quality time.

8. *The Referral Process*—Even though most people rely on their family physician during the referral process, the family physician may not always be the best referral source, and quite often the family physician does not know the best source for referral. The family physician will often refer patients to doctors within the geographical area or those that he or she knows through medical training or practice. Therefore, being aware of this shortcoming in the referral system is critical, taking into account that the family physician is usually the source for referral to a specialist.

A common three-stage referral approach most people take is (1) consultation with their family doctor; (2) referral, made by this same physician; and (3) making an appointment with a specialist. When a family experiences an illness or injury of an emergency nature, then panic, alienation, and fear set in. These feelings of panic, alienation, and fear are so overwhelming that it is very easy to put one hundred percent trust in the "rescuer" (the specialist physician), particularly because the family is most likely not expert on the particular medical problem and may have had no previous experience with medical emergencies. Undoubtedly, the family feels hope and comfort with the specialist. The specialist may be good but may not be the right physician for the medical problem.

## Importance of Selecting a Specialist or Subspecialist

Selecting a specialist is the *key* to increasing your chances of finding the right doctor. Even more important in our advanced medical profession is to use subspecialists. For example, in the case of a child's brain tumor, a specialist for surgically treating this condition would be the neurosurgeon. The subspecialty, therefore, would be the pediatric neurosurgeon. Childhood tumors are different from adult tumors in size, type, and growth characteristics. Therefore, the neurosurgeon tends to treat a wide spectrum of neurological problems that range from back, neck, hand, brain, and so forth, and most likely sees only a few cases of childhood brain tumors in his or her career. The pediatric neurosurgeon, by contrast, almost exclusively limits his or her practice to children and, therefore, will see many more of these cases. It is not uncommon for a busy pediatric neurosurgeon to see more childhood neurological cases in one year than some general neurosurgeons see in their entire medical career. Common sense tells us that the probability of a better result rests with the subspecialist. One can even argue that if a general neurosurgeon only performs one childhood brain tumor surgery per year, this physician will never be qualified to perform this type of surgery and should, therefore, automatically refer these cases to the pediatric neurosurgeon.

The case for pediatric care can be made for treatment of other childhood illnesses as well. In a special report on children's health care, *U.S. News & World Report* states,

> Unless the most imperiled of those children [children who are hospitalized for injuries or treated in emergency departments] are taken to a sophisticated children's hospital, or one especially geared for pediatric emergencies, the treatment they will receive is a crap shoot. Every day, some of America's children die, or almost die, because they are taken to the wrong hospital, treated with improper equipment, given wrong dosages of medications, or not diagnosed properly.[3]

As another example, let's examine the disease of arthritis. Dr. James Fries, director of the Stanford University Arthritis Clinic, reported that more than seventy-five million people in the United States experience joint and muscle pain and that more than three million suffer severe pain. Arthritis can be a totally disabling and life-threatening condition. A woman from Massachusetts had rheumatoid arthritis; her crippled and deformed fingers caused her severe, disabling pain. After conservative treatment failed, this woman finally found Dr. Alfred Swanson, a subspecialist orthopedist in Grand Rapids, Michigan, who specializes in finger joint replacement. Dr. Swanson successfully replaced the diseased joints of her fingers with tiny flexible silicone hinges. The procedure gave this patient restored mobility and eliminated her pain. Dr. Swanson reported that "out of the millions of Americans who potentially could benefit from the small joint implants, only about 200,000 have had surgery."[4] Many arthritic people suffer needlessly, consuming anti-inflammatory and pain medications when other options exist. This situation illustrates the importance of taking charge of your health care, seeking various options, and most important, finding a subspecialist for your medical problem.

Moreover, several different specialty areas may treat a particular disease. For example, orthopedics, neurosurgery, and plastic surgery may all treat hand problems. It is important that you investigate all of these options before making a treatment decision. For instance, a person with certain types of tendon disease in the hand may do better with a plastic surgeon than with an orthopedist or a neurosurgeon, owing to their particular type of training during residency. In summary, no matter what medical problem you are facing, a subspecialist will generally be more qualified than a regular specialist.

## Obtain an Accurate Diagnosis

Be sure that you have been given an accurate diagnosis. Major advances in diagnostic equipment have significantly aided in identifying medical problems. The advent of the CAT scan (Computer Axial Tomography), MRI (Magnetic

Resonance Imaging), PET scan (Petron-Emission Tomography), and more recently the MEG (Magnetoencephalography) have often made possible precise diagnoses. For example, as recently as a couple of decades ago, neurosurgeons were not able to adequately diagnose a brain tumor without first doing a biopsy. Today, through various examinations, surgeons are able to avoid unnecessary biopsies.

Even though the public, the government, and insurance companies bemoan the high cost of diagnostic tests and question their necessity, "medical products save millions of lives by detecting diseases before they spread, managing conditions that might otherwise threaten a life, or guiding a physician in conducting the most precise surgery possible."[5]

How can you assure yourself that you're getting the best diagnosis? It starts with selecting the right doctor, for it is the doctor who initiates the testing. A good doctor should complete a thorough exam that includes a detailed analysis of your past health, present symptoms, laboratory blood workup, physical examination, and a battery of tests. Surprisingly, some of the most common diagnostic errors result from a failure to complete one of these fundamentals. Failure of a complete diagnosis can result in missing a problem, diagnosing a nonexistent problem, substituting one problem for another, or failing to diagnose multiple causation.

For difficult cases, another way to help ensure an accurate diagnosis is to have a battery of tests conducted by a team of specialists. A general physician is not trained to be an expert in all disciplines as is a team of specialists from several specialty areas and will not be able to complete as thorough a diagnosis. If your medical problem is not defined and you find yourself going from doctor to doctor, you may begin to think that your pain is psychosomatic.

For example, one of the more recent evasive and difficult

illnesses to diagnose is lupus. Lupus is commonly one of two types: systemic and discoid erythematosus. Both are painful and potentially deadly inflammatory diseases. Several years ago a thirty-year-old woman was a happy and successful mother until she developed lingering fever with aches and pains all over her body, to the point where she had difficulty functioning. Doctors for months insisted that her problem was just emotional or was just a virus. Life became miserable as she continued to decline, until eventually her illness was diagnosed.[6] Many people face pain and suffering at the hands of physicians who can't accurately make a diagnosis or who refuse to use the medical system to help a patient reach a diagnosis.

If you have an undiagnosed or misdiagnosed illness, your chances for correct diagnosis are better if you consult a larger university medical center. These facilities utilize a team of specialists rather than just one specialty. To examine a patient, specialists depend largely upon their field of medicine. For example, pain in the chest area can be caused by a number of sources, such as the heart, ribs, muscles, esophagus, spine, shoulder, or digestive and other internal organs. The cardiologist will focus on the heart and circulatory system; while he or she might be able to exclude or rule out a heart problem, this patient is still left without a diagnosis. The neurologist may examine a person for this same condition and find that the pain is being caused by a pinched nerve in the spinal column that is producing a radiating pain from the spine to the chest area. In addition, there can be a combination of causes of pain in a given area. A person may have a mild heart condition of angina or pericarditis but also an undetected spinal tumor, or herniated disk. The cardiologist may treat only the heart condition to the exclusion of the primary disease in the spine. These multiple medical conditions can be more accurately detected by a good medical workup using a team of specialists. If you are being treated by a physician and continue to have pain and other symptoms, don't settle for evasive or ambiguous answers if your "gut" reaction and common sense suggests that something more is wrong.

## The Rule of Thumb—Get a Second Opinion

Most people are familiar with the axiom "Get a second opinion," especially if surgery is involved. There have been countless examples of misdiagnosis or poor surgical management. With the advances in medicine, medical problems can often be treated without surgery. Yet, fear will often affect our remembering this important step.

Another reason to seek a second opinion is to protect yourself against incompetent doctors, or outright bad treatment. For hundreds of years, literally thousands of books on quackery, promoting cure-all medicines from snake oil to tea leaves, have been sold. Dr. Victor Herbert, speaking at a cancer symposium, stated that "over 50,000 cancer patients a year have their health damaged and their pockets picked by promoters of nutrition quackery. Those most vulnerable to nutrition quackery are the many who are unable to distinguish genuine experts from charismatic snake oil salesmen." For example, he states that "Laetrile, a chemical derived from peach pits and long promoted as a cancer cure, is still over a billion-dollar industry despite studies published proving it is worthless."[7]

This is not to say that there are no useful nutritional diets and experts. With promising results, several valid studies and research projects are being conducted on the effects of vitamins in nutrition relative to cancer. At the same time, people must be aware of the quackery and harm that may result. This awareness is especially important when people face a terminal condition; they are extremely vulnerable and will often try anything in the hope of saving a life.

When consulting a physician for a second opinion, select a doctor who is not associated with the primary physician. If a neurosurgeon wants to operate, do not ask this doctor for a referral, because you stand the chance of being referred to his or her associate or indirect associate. There may be a tendency for a consulting neurosurgeon to agree with the referring neurosurgeon because of professional courtesy, similar practice patterns, or indirect monetary incentives through continued referrals, peer review pressures, or business association. Many surgeons will request that you obtain a second opinion from an associate; this associate will most likely agree with your surgeon, thereby justifying the need for surgery. *Prior to any surgery, you should obtain multiple, unbiased opinions.* The more extensive the planned surgery, the more opinions you should receive. Also consult a doctor who is not a surgeon, because nonsurgeons may offer alternative treatments.

## Obtain Your Records

Prior to visiting the consulting doctor, bring all appropriate medical records. These records may consist of previous operating reports, office chart notes, history and physical reports, laboratory and pathologist reports, radiologist reports, and original pre- and post-X-ray and other diagnostic films. The original diagnostic films are generally better than a copy because they are genuinely clearer. Also, most surgeons prior to performing surgery will want to view the diagnostic films and will not rely on a radiologist's written report. A doctor's office may tell you that you are not allowed to have the X-rays, reports, and so forth, or even copies. This should be a warning sign to you that the doctor may be "territorial" and not willing to let go of patients even if the patients might be better served elsewhere. The law states, however, that you are entitled to copies of everything in your patient file (though you may have to pay a fee for the copies).

Package all this information in a well-organized and chronological fashion to help the consulting doctor formulate an opinion more easily. Although second opinions are best completed in person, you can mail the entire package along with a cover letter to a doctor and receive an opinion by telephone or mail. Many doctors do not charge for this service, but a written consultation report is generally not prepared.

# 2

# Starting Your Search
# —Ten Sources

*You don't have to be an expert* on the medical problem, but you do need to educate yourself as much as possible on the disease, treatment alternatives, and medical facilities. Later, when you are ready to begin your networking process (chapter 5), you will already have a list of potential sources and doctors. Explained below are ten basic sources to begin the process of educating yourself.

1. *Your local doctor, hospital, and staff*—Ask as many questions as you can about the problem of your family physician, his staff, and hospital personnel. Become familiar with the terminology for your particular medical problem. Understand the basic physiology and description of the problem. The more you know about the problem, the better you will later be able to converse with doctors about their opinions. As Don Quixote said, "The beginning of health is to know the disease." When talking with your doctor, remember that there is no such thing as a stupid question. *Any question is better than no question at all.* Once you begin to ask questions, dialogue will generally follow and additional questions will naturally emerge. Ask your doctor to explain the disease to you in simple terms. Ask your doctor for patient guides, office medical books, medical encyclopedias and other medical literature and research articles that he

or she may have available in the office. Geigy Pharmaceuticals, a division of CIBA-Geigy, produces booklets called "Clinical Symposia" that review specific diseases in easy-to-understand language with many colorful illustrations. If the doctor doesn't have enough time to teach you, ask if his or her assistant can help you. Use medical staff members and the information they give you to help you sift through and understand medical jargon and technical terminology.

2. *Medical libraries*—Go to a medical library and spend time reading the medical encyclopedia, journals, and articles on the subject. If you have a child or family member who has been admitted to a hospital for tests, spend your time in the hospital's medical library rather than sitting in the waiting room and worrying. Learning about the disease will allow you to ask your doctor more intelligent questions about treatment options and how to manage and cope with the disease. For example, if you want to find out who is one of the best thoracic surgeons, look in the medical journals to see who is doing the research and scientific studies on thoracic surgery. Likewise, if the problem involves plastic surgery, rheumatology, or urology, look up these topics in the journals and find out which people are doing the research in these areas. These doctors will later be excellent contacts and may themselves end up being the right doctor for you. Ask the librarian for assistance in running a computer search of the particular topic.

3. *Newspaper clippings, or articles*—Be alert for medical articles that appear in magazines and newspapers. These sources often publish stories about major breakthroughs in medicine. Use the names of any doctors mentioned in the articles to contact later on when you begin your networking process.

Call or write the people mentioned in the article to learn more about their situation and how it may be similar to yours. However, be sure that the story is authentic and not hyped. Also, some medical facilities' reputations can be built upon the amount of media they receive. Your judgment of a facility can also be jaded by previous publicity, such as the past pioneering of a new procedure or scientific break-through.

4. *Medical hotlines*—Hotline services provide names of physicians, treatment protocols, and counseling. One example of a hotline service is the Surgical Opinion Hotline set up by the U.S. government for citizens to obtain names of physicians to contact for second opinions (1-800-638-6833). Other hotlines are available for substance abuse dependency, AIDS, and so on. Hotline services are becoming widespread but are limited in their information because they may not have all the names of the best doctors and latest treatments. The names of the physicians included in their databases are often only those doctors who are associated with the hotline organization. Still, hotline services can be a very quick, immediate method to get you started in your search. Each hotline varies in the amount of information it provides, but most are generally able to send you literature, treatment options, and a list of physicians in your area.

A listing of hotline numbers and sources are listed in the appendix.

5. *Consulting groups*—Medical consulting groups are becoming more popular and sophisticated. These agencies, for a fee, will provide up-to-date clinical information and network services. One such group, the Cancer Consulting Group (1-312-866-7711), located in Evanston, Illinois, specializes in cancer. The group provides information about cancer and its treatments, conducts research among a network of experts, and answers questions. The appendix includes various consulting groups.

Local hospitals are beginning to offer free consultations

with their local doctors. This source can be valuable, but remember that the doctor is likely to steer you toward other doctors within the same hospital. Consulting groups are very limited; therefore, your search should not be limited to this source.

6. *Computer database systems*—Computer database systems are breaking into the medical profession and can be a significant help in your search. The National Cancer Institute utilizes a system called the PDQ (Physicians Data Query, 1-800-422-6232, which allows physicians to tie into the PDQ system and access state-of-the-art information on the diagnosis and treatment of cancer. It also provides the public with names of experts, experimental therapies, and institutions. Dr. Vincent T. DeVita, Jr., states, "This is the largest informational database of its kind, and if used widely, could save thousands of additional lives per year."[8]

Another computer database system is the Health Resource Company (1-502-329-5272), which provides both mini- and lengthy reports from the lay and medical press on specific medical conditions. This computer search comprises information from medical journals, newspapers, organizations, magazine articles, and so forth.

Though computer database systems are very limited and charge fees for their use, they may not always be up to date. Therefore, use the information as a springboard during your networking process. A listing of various computer database systems is included in Appendix C.

7. *Talk to others who have had a similar problem*—Talk to people who have had a similar medical problem. You might ask hospital personnel or your doctor for names. They can be excellent sources for referral. These people can also be especially valuable in helping you deal with treatment and post-treatment recovery and can offer you valuable advice.

Often you can avoid the same mistakes that others have made and can capitalize on their experience.

8. *Physician referral services*—Most major cities have physician referral services that are either privately or publicly operated and are designed to provide names of local doctors in various specialties. Most of these services are free of charge, although some require a fee. Many are operated by hospitals. These services can have drawbacks. They usually are limited to physicians of a local area or hospital affiliation, or to those doctors who have paid a fee to have their names listed. Also, some of the services may not carefully scrutinize the doctors' credentials. These services can be helpful but are not always reliable.

9. *Associations*—There are many good associations, and they can often be your best source of information about available treatment, support groups, research information, and, most important, directories of specialists and treatment centers. They also are often a good source for up-to-date treatment information and cutting-edge treatment, but they do have their drawbacks as well. They are limited to the quality of their volunteers, personnel, and funding, and they can be influenced by their medical directors, boards, and the legal environment. Also, not every illness or disease may have an association. They do not make referrals or give medical advice and information, especially if the treatment is experimental. For this reason, many associations tend to restrict their referrals to large, well-established medical universities and teaching hospitals. Appendix A lists categories of illnesses and medical conditions, along with related associations' addresses and phone numbers.

10. *Surveys of top doctors and hospitals*—The use of surveys listing the top medical doctors or medical facilities can be a tremendous asset in your search campaign. However, it is more important to understand how to go

about using the surveys than to take the survey results as absolute and thereby exclude other doctors and facilities. Surveys are generally conducted on the telephone by a researcher and sometimes followed up with personal interviews or through the use of questionnaires. The researcher's population is generally a few hundred (or in some cases up to 1000 or more) doctors and/or hospital administrators. The survey asks their opinions about various doctors or medical facilities. Typical questions are these: "To whom would you turn in case of your own illness?" or "Which medical facility is the best for treating a specific medical problem?"

Surveys can have limitations. They often are not true indicators of the best doctors or medical facilities. First, the criteria used—asking a limited population of doctors or hospital administrators—may not be valid. The ranking of the doctors is often done solely on the basis of frequency. In other words, the doctors selected the most often would receive the most points and consequently have the higher ranking.

Second, many doctors may never make the list simply because they are not well-known. Reputations of doctors and hospitals are often made through quantity of research publications and media exposure. It is easier to assess a doctor's knowledge through his academic abilities (i.e., publishing) than through actual technical skills. A highly skilled doctor might not publish. Likewise, an academic doctor who publishes considerably may not be the best, most skilled doctor.

Third, respondents can also be influenced by the preexisting reputation of doctors or facilities, especially those that have been around for a long time and are well established. Doctors have different opinions on whether their practice should be marketed. A young, brilliant doctor who is very skillful may not be widely known, especially if he or she is starting a new specialty program. If the doctor does not promote his or her practice through public relations, the doctor's efforts may not be widely known. In addition, some doctors or medical facilities who had a fine reputation years ago may not now be as good.

John Pekkanen, in his survey, "The Best Medical Specialists in the U.S.," states,

> Certainly not every outstanding physician in this country is listed in a survey. There are literally tens of thousands of them. Many don't come to national recognition because they do not publish widely, or belong to national medical organizations, or do other things where they come to the attention of, and are evaluated by, their peers.[9]

Dr. Herbert Dietrich states in regard to his own survey, *The Best in Medicine*, "Keep in mind that institutions not appearing in this list of hospitals and clinics rated for overall excellence may, in certain specialties, be quite comparable to or even surpass those that are listed."[10]

Even with their limitations, surveys can be your most powerful networking source, depending upon how you use them. Don't rely on the rankings of the survey as absolute. This is a critical point. Remember it! Use the survey only as a networking tool to find the best doctor or facility through your questioning techniques as you call the people on the survey. Appendix D provides a comprehensive survey from *U.S. News & World Report*. Appendix E lists other survey sources.

## How to Improve Your Results—Self-Management

How can you improve the results of your search for information, doctors, and treatments? Attitude and skills are two key ingredients necessary for a successful search campaign. You need to be confident. Know what you want to accomplish (attitude) and how you are going to achieve it (skills). Following are several principles and methods that will help you improve your results in your search campaign:

1. *Manage it yourself*—You must accept the fact that you are going to be conducting your search campaign yourself. Don't rely on your family physician, medical specialist, or local hospital. Finding the right doctor, particularly for a serious medical problem, can be almost a full-time job. Therefore, you must put time aside and make it happen yourself. For example, you may want to devote a period of time each day to work on it, such as during your lunch hour or before or after work.

2. *Get help*—Talk to all you meet—family members, strangers, or friends—and ask for their help. Many people and agencies are willing to lend a hand. Enlisting many people working on the same task can produce significantly higher results. Consult and join associations specializing in your illness.

3. *Imagination and initiative*—People should have imagination and creativity and try different routes and avenues not commonly used. Instead of just relying on your local hospital, look to other institutions. There may be a specialist in your own area who has the expertise you are looking for. Nevertheless, don't be afraid to reach out. If you live in California, don't hesitate to consult the Southwest, Midwest, or East. We live in a jet age in which we can literally fly anywhere in the country in a few hours. Take advantage of this option.

4. *Information is power*—Do your homework. The more information you acquire, the more power you add to your search. Understanding the medical problem will allow you to talk more intelligently with doctors, explore alternatives, and arrive at an effective decision.

5. *Hard work*—Be prepared for a great deal of physical, mental, and emotional hard work. It is not easy to conduct a search campaign.

6. *Ask the right questions*—Learn to ask the appropriate questions of the doctor. Prepare these questions in advance. We will explore the art of good questions in chapter 5.

7. *Develop a referral network*—You will improve your chances of finding the right doctor if you can develop a contact or referral system. If you are able to obtain a doctor's name as a reference from your present doctor, it is more likely that you will get to talk to the specialist. Find good "lead-ins" and avenues to make entry in talking to your specialist. As a rule of thumb, it is easier to talk to someone if you have a contact.

8. *Dedication and confidence*—Seneca once said, "Lack of confidence is not the result of difficulty; the difficulty comes from lack of confidence." Believe in yourself; don't let fate take over. Don't complain, sulk, or resign yourself that you are not getting anywhere. Keep going!

9. *Use the telephone*—The telephone can be a more convenient and quick way to correspond with specialists than writing letters or visiting personally.

10. *The 80/20 rule*—People frequently spend too much time on activities that do not work toward achieving their goals. The 80/20 rule states that eighty percent of one's time is spent on nonessential activities and only twenty percent on the essentials. For example, you might spend too much time talking about how the problem happened instead of what you're going to do about it. Remember this rule.

11. *Take good notes and write down all discussions*— During every discussion, whether in person or on the telephone, you should record everything. This will help you later to analyze your information and make a final decision.

12. *Avoid procrastination*—Become self-motivated and

get started. In most cases, it can be helpful to set deadlines and reasonable time frames. Keep in mind, though, that "overplanning" can also be a form of procrastination.

13. *Think before you act*—Prior to initiating a telephone call, you should plan what you are going to say and how you are going to say it. Write it down and rehearse it. Make your questions and statements clear and to the point.

14. *"To Do" list*—Develop a "To Do" list, writing and prioritizing (A, B, C) the activities that you want to accomplish to meet your goals. "A" items are the highest priority, and you should start on them first. "B" items are the next priority, and "C" items are the lowest priority items. Complete the "A" priority items before working on the "B" and "C" priority items.

Also, cross off each activity as you complete it. Continue to prioritize your activities as you progress. Figure 2-1 presents an example of a practical "To Do" list.

15. *Keep praying*—Never stop praying. God heals through prayer. Prayer provides an in-depth communication with God. Pray for strength, courage, direction, and healing. Healing can take place instantly or gradually. Dr. Ben Carson, director of pediatric neurosurgery at Johns Hopkins University Hospital, cites in his book *Think Big*, several miracles by God when Carson was at the operating table. For example, once while operating inside a brain, an artery broke, resulting in uncontrolled bleeding, and Dr. Carson pleaded, "God, you've got to stop the bleeding. Please, God! I cannot control it." Dr. Carson stated, "At that instant the bleeding stopped without my being able to locate its cause."[11] An entire book could be written just on the stories of healing miracles obtained through prayer. Throughout our own national media exposure, we have received hundreds of phone calls from across the country and heard many testimonies about the power of prayer.

*"To Do" Health List*

| A,B,C | Activity | Date Completed |
|---|---|---|
| A | Call Doctor Smith | |
| A | Start Referral Network | |
| C | Read Articles in Medical Library | |
| B | Visit Special Medical Center | |
| A | Call Hotline | |
| C | Call Hospital | |
| C | Call Relative | |
| C | Write Referral Letters | |
| A | Get Medical Survey from Jim | |
| C | Get copies of x-ray and MRI files | |
| B | Join Association | |
| | | |
| | | |
| | | |
| | | |

**Figure 2–1 A Practical Health "To Do" List
for Managing Your Networking Activities**

# 3

# Understanding
# the Medical System

## The Financial Side of Taking Charge

*Taking charge financially of your medical care* requires an understanding of the inner workings of the health-care industry. The total national health-care expenditure now exceeds 600 billion dollars per year (14% of the GNP), and nearly one quarter of this amount is paid directly by you, the consumer.

A significant factor that determines the quality of your health care is the type of health-insurance coverage you have. Finding the best doctor for your medical problem is largely dependent on whether or not your health-insurance plan allows freedom of choice in doctor selection. Therefore, you should understand your health-insurance coverage before you begin your search. Even more important, you should select the best health-insurance plan from a cost-benefit standpoint *prior* to experiencing a life-threatening illness.

The major types of health plans today are Medicare, Medicaid, private carrier, health maintenance organizations (HMO), preferred provider organizations (PPO), worker compensation, and special government programs.

*Medicare* presently serves about thirteen percent of all

123

people in the United States and is federally funded by the Health Care Financing Administration (HCFA). It is offered to people who are at least sixty-five years old; other eligible people are long-term disabled, and railroad retirees. The program has two parts—Medicare Part A and Medicare Part B. Part A covers hospital-related expenses such as the room, meals, medications, and skilled hospital personnel. The Part B plan covers items such as the doctor's fees, outpatient diagnostic and laboratory testing, and durable medical equipment.

Prior to enrolling in Medicare, thoroughly investigate this program and compare it with other available plans. Talk to local hospital-insurance administrators, insurance agents, and the Social Security Office. You can receive literature from your local Social Security Office, American Association of Retired Persons (AARP), and your state medical associations, all of which will help you determine if Medicare is right for you.

Even though Medicare may offer the lowest monthly premium, you need to understand some of the limitations to this program. The biggest limitation in working with Medicare is that it is like playing old Chinese baseball. When you hit the ball, you never know where to run, since the players are allowed to move the bases. Likewise, Medicare is constantly changing the rules, and patients and doctors never know from one day to the next what the rules are. There can be constant frustration and confusion in keeping up with these rules. Many rules are very ambiguous, making it difficult for medical providers to understand them and know how to operate their practices. Many doctors have stayed away from Medicare because of the large amount of paperwork, constant changes, threats of fines, regular audits, low reimbursement schedules, higher incidence of refiling claim forms, prior-approval regulations, flat service fees for hospitals, and medical service restrictions.

For example, a Medicare patient suffered from a serious joint disease, and the surgeon recommended a custom-made implant (prosthesis). Prior to the patient's admission, the hospital determined that it would lose a substantial amount of money to do the procedure based upon the flat fee Medicare would pay the hospital. This flat fee, known as the Diagnostic Related Group (DRG), is based upon average length of stay for each diagnosis. More disturbing to the patient was the fact that the cost of the prosthesis alone was nearly the entire DRG fee. When the hospital refused to allow the procedure, the patient requested that she be allowed to pay the difference, an amount that she was very willing and able to pay. However, according to Medicare guidelines, this is illegal. The patient suffered until she finally found a facility that allowed the procedure, but she had a less qualified surgeon than the one she had originally selected. Examples like this are typical and have led some people to feel that the Medicare program creates added stress and frustration, shorter hospital stays, lower-quality products and services, and hospital closings.

*Medicaid* represents eighteen percent of all plans and is a federal government health-insurance program that is administered by each state. Both the federal and state governments share in the cost of the program. This plan is available for low-income people and is especially good for people who have suffered an unexpected hardship such as loss of a job or life-threatening illness. Its guidelines vary from state to state, although generally eligibility is based upon income, assets, and family size.

Though the Medicaid patient does not pay anything for medical services, neither is the Medicaid program without limitations. Some of the limitations include a limited reimbursement schedule for providers, government audits, restrictions on services, and overall greater paperwork in processing insurance claims. In addition, one of the unfortunate limitations for the Medicaid patient is the low regard that many health professionals hold of Medicaid patients. Some doctors and other health professionals view Medicaid patients as more troublesome, less healthy, more prone to sickness, less apt to care for themselves, and more likely to complain. Whether or not this is true, many physicians do not become Medicaid providers, thereby limiting the number of available doctors. Therefore, the Medicaid patient may have difficulty finding the best or most desired doctor. In addition, Medicaid patients are restricted to using doctors within their state.

*Private health-insurance plans* are considered to be best, in terms of comprehensive coverage and with the lowest number of restrictions and bureaucracy for the physician and hospital. However, many of these traditional plans have gone through their own streamlining and cost controls. While the best plans are highly valued by the medical provider, many companies are finding them too costly to offer to their employees; therefore, the best plans are generally found only with profitable corporations. As with all plans, read the policy carefully, particularly such phrases as preexisting medical problems, prior approvals, high deductibles, low-maximum lifetime premium amounts, and doctor selection.

*Health Maintenance Organizations (HMOs)* began in the early 1960s and have grown to approximately 300 different companies representing more than ten million people. HMOs were originally designed to keep costs down and maintain quality care, with emphasis on preventive health care. There are many types of HMOs, such as independent practice associations and social HMOs, all having a variety of advantages and disadvantages. In most of these plans, the member pays a one-time fee (commonly called pay-as-you-go) and does not pay a deductible. While many of these plans have worked well, many have had their difficulties; you need to be very careful and to understand your individual plan.

Sometimes, services are restricted to your own geographical area, require prior approval or authorizations, and have limitations on the facilities and doctors you select. Another criticism is that some HMOs are physician-owned and controlled, so their remuneration is dependent on their ability to contain costs. In such HMOs, physicians may be reluctant to order diagnostic tests or to refer the patient to a specialist. *Medical Economics* reported that "financial incentives to manipulate physician behavior are as old as HMOs ... A number of recent lawsuits have charged that such financial incentives induced doctors to deny lifesaving tests or referrals—however, no suit has proved a causal connection."[12]

Overall, however, there are some very good HMOs, and several have recently started employing quality-of-care measures and stricter quality-care audits. For more information, write to the Group Health Association of America at 1717 Massachusetts Ave. NW, Washington, DC 20036.

*Preferred Provider Organizations (PPO)* are another type of health-insurance plan that works on the principle of keeping costs down by limiting you to only "preferred" providers. Failure to use one of these preferred providers may result in a much higher deductible (penalty), a bigger co-payment, or *exclusion from any coverage at all.* This drawback is of major concern if you need a subspecialist not on the list of preferred providers.

*Worker Compensation* insurance plans generally provide excellent coverage, but of course these insurance plans are purchased by employers and are limited to employee work injuries. Although aspects of these plans are regulated by the state, they can have their limitations as well. Patients are often caught up in legal disputes and years of litigation while the court determines if the claim is valid. Other times, since the employee is being paid while off work, the patient may be reluctant to return to work and therefore abuses the program. The patient may also not be allowed to be treated by the doctor of his or her choice because in many states the compensation carrier is allowed to select the doctor. In order to monitor the course of treatment, which scrutiny some patients find uncomfortable, some compensation carriers hire professional nurse consultants. Some carriers will also make a final lump settlement based upon the patient's permanent partial impairment (PPI) rating, leaving the patient with perhaps no further insurance coverage for the specific injury.

*Other special government plans* include CHAMPUS and VA plans. CHAMPUS is designed for active and retired military personnel and families, and VA coverage is for veterans of war. CHAMPUS operates similarly to HMOs but without service fees. VA coverage, which serves about three million patients, is also free but is restricted to government VA hospitals. Your selection of physician is limited, and you may not always get the same physician. Also, the VA hospital system is often hampered by inadequate government funding. The VA hospital system, which comprises 171 hospitals, includes some hospitals affiliated with teaching facilities. You may have better-quality care with one of these larger teaching-affiliated VA hospitals.

*Self-pay*, or having no insurance at all, is one of the most difficult positions one can be in when faced with a life-threatening illness. One out of every five Americans (37 million) does not have health insurance, and an estimated ninety million Americans have inadequate coverage. This is a difficult position, but there are options to enable you to receive medical care. You should first start by talking to the social services department of your area hospital. These people can generally direct you to special financial aid services. Many hospitals have special indigent plans for which you may qualify. For example, the Hill-Burton Hospital Free Care Program is available for people meeting specific requirements. Call 1-800-638-0742 to receive information about hospitals participating in this program. The Shriners Hospital system is another source of free care for children under eighteen who need orthopedic or burn treatment. Call 1-800-237-5055 for information.

In addition, many physicians will perform their services for free or for a reduced fee. County hospitals often provide special help for in-county residents, and university teaching medical schools will sometimes take on these (hardship) cases. Special fundraising events and charitable organizations can provide much if not all of the financial needs for medical care and should not be overlooked.

Lastly, people who resign or are terminated from their jobs should investigate enrolling in the COBRA (Consolidated Omnibus Budget Reconciliation Act) plan. Under federal law, employers are required to permit ex-employees to remain in their health-insurance program at least eighteen months and possibly up to three years; the ex-employee must pay full premiums and must sign up within sixty days after leaving the job.

With some serious diseases, many people find that most of their savings eventually become exhausted; they may then be eligible for Medicaid and other special government and charitable assistance programs. Some treatments, when possible, may be prolonged until the patient can qualify for assistance such as Medicaid or welfare.

If your medical problem is one for which there is not yet a standard treatment procedure, you might consider contacting the National Institutes of Health (NIH). The NIH is research-oriented and conducts clinical studies of new types of treatment. Therefore, a patient selected for treatment by the NIH does not have to pay for services. If current treatment is not generally successful for the medical problem, a patient may benefit from trying a new treatment. Contact the NIH at 301-496-4891 or by writing:

> Office of the Director
> The Clinical Center
> Building 10, Room 2C-146
> National Institutes of Health
> Bethesda, MD 20892

## Cutting Financial Corners—Cost-Saving Strategies

Several cost-saving strategies can be utilized when conducting your search. The following are cost-saving strategies that can help you save money.

1. *Accept Insurance (AI)*—If you are in a tight financial situation with mounting bills and a reduced income, consider asking the doctor if he or she will accept insurance. "Accept insurance" means that the physician agrees to take the insurance payment as full payment for services rendered without requiring you to pay the balance. The physician's office refers to this type of patient account as an "AI" account and will write off the balance of your account. Even though the physician may accept insurance payment in full without requiring you to pay the balance, it is not considered legal for the physician to advertise this procedure for all patients. Moreover, many insurance plans require the physician to make a reasonable effort to collect the balance of the payment from the patient, yet many physicians will accept insurance for selected patients. Some medical providers may provide incentives for cash payments; others may try to

restrict these practices in order to be consistent and prevent widespread use by all patients.

2. *Reasonable and Customary Fees*—It is to your advantage if the medical provider accepts "usual, customary, and reasonable" fees (UCR). This rate is the average fee charged for procedures or services in the geographical area of the provider. If your provider charges a higher fee than the reasonable and customary rate indicated on the "Explanation of Benefits" (EOB) health-insurance payment form, then you will not be responsible for any amount above this rate. Though most providers agree to accept this rate, it is important that you inquire about this ahead of time.

3. *Discuss the diagnostic testing in advance*—The decision to order diagnostic testing can have an important financial impact. Diagnostic testing is often an abused area of medical health care. Prior to undergoing any diagnostic or laboratory test, you should understand exactly why the test is necessary and how often it needs to be performed. Among physicians, wide differences exist in the frequency and number of tests ordered. Some physicians may run unnecessary tests to protect themselves legally in case of potential malpractice suits or for documentation in personal injury cases. Other physicians, to help contribute to their medical facility's profitability, may feel pressure from their medical facility to order tests.

Not all tests may be as important as others in diagnosing your disease. For example, if you have severe low-back pain, a number of diagnostic tests could be ordered, such as X-rays, MRI, CAT, EMG, Doppler, myelogram, and so forth. Each of these tests can provide unique information. However, running all these tests, especially early in your medical care, may be unnecessary and costs thousands of dollars. By utilizing just X-rays and MRI, the physician may be able to make a diagnosis. Dr. John Egerton states, "Sometimes we spend a great deal of money unneccessarily by seeking a definitive diagnosis. We may look to confirm a clinical opinion or rule out some unlikely disease, perhaps to reassure either the patient or ourselves. In many cases, however, we could avoid the expensive tests and serve our patients just as well."[13]

Some tests may be ordered to confirm a diagnosis, but the course of treatment may be the same anyway. For the physician, some information can be "nice to know," while other information is critical. Also, some tests simply have more risks than others. You should always ask the doctor why the test is being ordered and if alternative tests are available. Ask the doctor about the likelihood of the proposed test's providing the necessary diagnostic information and about the risks involved for the test as compared to other tests. For example, the myelogram is an invasive test in which the physician injects dye into the spinal cord fluid with a needle. This test can cause more complications for the patient than undergoing a simple MRI scan.

There also may be underlying financial incentives for the physician to run a certain test. A physician may desire that you undergo at his or her facility the same test that you may have just completed elsewhere. Likewise, some physicians may order certain laboratory blood tests even though the same tests may have to be redone prior to surgery because of hospital policy. Other times, the physician may run a battery of blood tests when perhaps he or she could get by with running only a few basic laboratory tests first to see if the values are normal or not. If abnormal values are obtained, then additional tests can be run. Yet, some doctors may fail to obtain even the most basic tests indicated for making a diagnosis or prior to administering treatment.

Understand the purpose and frequency of tests prior to undergoing them. Don't be afraid to question your doctor. It may not only save much time, pain, potential complications, and side effects, but your pocketbook as well.

4. *Know your insurance policy coverage*—Prior to undergoing any diagnostic procedure or treatment, study your insurance policy and coverages, exclusions, and exemptions. This can save you from a large and unexpected bill. Don't take for granted that the medical provider will do this for you. Many policies may have penalties for failure to obtain prior approval, or for not using certain "preferred" providers. Check the limits of maximum coverage for your health-insurance policy. Consider the deductible that you yourself have to pay. Once this is met, you may want to undergo treatment or testing before the end of the year, before the deductible starts all over again the next year.

5. *Supplemental Insurance Coverages*—Always brainstorm for possible insurance coverage through supplemental policies, such as your spouse's plan, homeowner's plan, automobile insurance, or worker's compensation coverage. These plans can be especially useful in case of accidents.

If you should lose your job, you may not have to lose your health insurance. As discussed previously, companies are required by law under the COBRA government guidelines to permit an ex-employee to pay for continued health-insurance coverage for eighteen months after termination (unless termination was for disciplinary reasons). Check with your personnel office for information on COBRA.

6. *Assignment of Benefits*—Consider medical providers who permit assignment of benefits. This is an agreement between the provider and your health-insurance company to pay the provider directly. You won't have to pay the medical provider first and then have to file a claim with your insurance company for reimbursement. You are only required to pay your portion after the medical provider has received the insurance payment. Many months can pass

before you have to pay your portion. All it may take to activate this process is your simple signature in the medical provider's office indicating your agreement for transfer or "assignment of benefits."

7. *Cash Payments*—In some cases, the medical provider may offer financial incentives if you pay cash for your services. Some medical providers may also significantly reduce your overall account balance if you pay a lump cash sum to avoid long-term collections and credit bureaus. Don't be afraid to ask your medical provider about cash payments.

8. *Claim Denial Appeals*—Just because your health-insurance claim has been denied, does not mean you are stuck with the bill. Insurance claims may be rejected because they were not correctly filled out by the medical provider, and they may simply need to be refiled. Also, if a procedure was more extensive than originally predicted, the physician may need to include a special billing code modifier, or write a supporting letter stating the necessity for the extensive procedure and higher fee. Consult your health-insurance supervisor or manager and learn exactly the details of your billing situation.

9. *Keep track of all expenditures*—Take time to read and understand the listing of all medical services, procedures, and supplies utilized. Medical providers do make mistakes and can bill you for services not rendered. Keep good records and save all your receipts for tax deductions.

10. *Other Medical Expenses*—Ask the doctor if prescribed therapeutic aids, physical therapy, or durable medical equipment (such as braces, electrical stimulators, or hospital beds) are absolutely necessary. Be aware that a good source of revenue for a hospital or for a doctor derives from prescribing ancillary services, such as physical therapy or durable medical equipment. If a treatment is deemed absolutely necessary, do not hesitate to price-shop. For

example, a simple TENS unit (electrical stimulator for pain) can range from $200 to $800 for the same unit.

11. *Train family members to provide care*—Many services can be provided by family members without hiring high-cost professionals. The doctor may be able to teach you or a family member to give injections, change dressings, and provide physical and rehabilitative therapy. This can be especially cost-effective for long-term illnesses. Too, there are several self-help courses available through local hospitals and Red Cross agencies. Volunteer organizations such as the Arthritis and Diabetes Foundations also provide free services and self-help instruction.

12. *Prescriptions*—Chances are that you are going to be given medicine prescriptions. More than two billion dollars of prescription drugs are sold annually, with over 400,000 prescription drugs now available. Since most physicians receive free drug samples from drug companies, ask the doctor for these complimentary samples. Or, ask the doctor to substitute the generic version of the drug; generic drugs are often similar in quality but at a much lower cost. Also, price-shop pharmacies; prices for the same drug vary widely.

In addition to being price-conscious, learn as much as you can about the drugs you are required to take. Besides your doctor, pharmacists are excellent sources of information, cost differences, comparable drugs, adverse reaction comparisons, new drugs, and so on. It has been reported that approximately forty percent of medication users experience undesirable side effects.[14] These side effects can be reduced by learning about the drug, other drug options, and methods to reduce those side effects unique to your condition. Appendix F lists several references for learning about prescription drugs.

## Patient Rights and Services

The relationship between you and your doctor is a two-way street and is important to the quality of your care. Both you and your doctor should have mutual respect for each other. When this relationship ceases to exist, it's time either to rectify the situation or find another doctor. The Patient Bill of Rights, adopted by the American Hospital Association, provides several guidelines for you in understanding your rights as a patient. A copy of these rights can be found in Appendix H.

The more important rights relate to medical information, the consent form, and patient confidentiality and privacy. As discussed in chapter 1, you are entitled to all the medical information concerning your care and can receive copies of your records upon written notice. The medical provider is allowed to charge you a reasonable fee for copies of your records. If you are getting a second opinion, the medical provider may allow you to borrow the original X-ray films, although many medical providers attempt to charge you for a copy rather than release the original.

Prior to signing a consent form, be sure that you understand all the information necessary to make an intelligent decision. The medical provider should explain radiology reports, diagnostic films, laboratory reports, and so forth. You may also want to view videotapes and literature on the procedure prior to signing the consent form. *Never sign a blank consent form and allow the doctor to fill it in at a later time.* You may also want to have a third-party witness, such as a relative or health professional, help you understand the proposed medical procedure. This method can help legally protect both you and the doctor by ensuring that the doctor explained the alternative treatment options, risks, and proposed details of the procedure, and that you understood this information.

Regarding the issue of confidentiality and privacy, *never allow your medical records to be given to anyone without your written permission.* The medical provider has the fiduciary responsibility to keep your medical file private. Releasing this information could jeopardize your chances for future job openings, enrolling in health- and life-insurance programs, personal injury cases, political activities, and so on. The ownership of your records generally belongs to the files of your medical provider, but you have the right to dictate where copies of this information goes. Medical providers are required by law to maintain your medical files for five to seven years, generally, depending upon state law.

# 4

# Avoiding the Wrong Doctor

*As you begin your search* for the "right" doctor, you must also be concerned with avoiding the "wrong" doctor. Between 1970 and 1988, the number of physicians increased by 75 percent, reaching nearly 600,000 physicians nationally. The number of specialties has significantly increased as well. All these physicians are not going to have the same degree of skills or talent. An estimated five to ten percent of physicians annually are deemed incompetent because of alcohol, drugs, or mental health impairment.[15] Therefore, how can you be sure that your doctor is competent?

## The Health Care Quality Improvement Act

Fortunately, federal laws are helping to weed out incompetent doctors by imposing reporting requirements on medical-care institutions, health boards, medical societies, and physicians. The Health Care Quality Improvement Act of 1986 (Title IV of P.L. 99–660) established the National Practitioner Data Bank to hinder incompetent doctors from moving from state to state, by exposing their prior misconduct or substandard care record. The data in the National Practitioner Data Bank are not available to the general public; the Privacy Act protects the physicians' information from public disclosure. As health consumers, however, we can be assured that hospitals and other health-care entities are required by law to utilize the information in the Data Bank. Hospitals and other health-care entities, prior to granting clinical staff privileges to a physician, must request from the Data Bank the file report on the applying physician. The intent of releasing this information is to assist the hospital in screening the applicants and rejecting incompetent physicians. Hospitals and other health-care entitities are also required to request the file reports every two years for all medical staff physicians.

The law further requires that medical professional societies, hospitals and other health-care entities, and state medical boards must report to the Data Bank any disciplinary actions taken against a physician. These actions include any improper professional conduct that adversely affects the physician's medical license, clinical privileges, or membership in medical organizations. Medical malpractice insurance carriers are also required to report to state medical licensing boards monetary payments made on claims against a physician for settlement of a malpractice claim or judgment. In addition, individual physicians are required to declare any self-insured payments made on their own behalf for any malpractice suit.

The purpose of the National Practitioner Data Bank is not to render against a physician a negative judgment based on the number of malpractice claims filed against the physician. In our highly litigious society, it is not unusual for a very competent physician, especially in the specialty areas of orthopedics, obstetrics, or neurosurgery, to have several malpractice claims. An out-of-court settlement of a malpractice claim, which is often out of the control of the physician, does not necessarily indicate wrongdoing or incompetence. It may be more a factor of the physician's specialty area, frequency of complicated cases, personal risk tolerance, or the propensity for malpractice suits in the area. Even though the information in the Data Bank is not accessible to the general public, most state medical licensing agencies or attorneys general offices will provide information about physicians regarding disciplinary actions and a number of malpractice claims.

More information on the Data Bank can be received from the Division of Quality Assurance and Liability Management, Bureau of Health Professions, U.S. Department of Health and Human Services, in Washington, D.C., or from the Data Bank Help Line at 1-800-767-6732.

As a practical matter, be on the alert for medical practice patterns that appear unusual, such as physicians who practice without hospital privileges, operate their own centers without any affiliation to area hospitals, or offer exotic treatments. If the physician operates out of his or her own surgery clinic, verify that the physician has not been relieved of hospital staff privileges. Don't be afraid to ask a doctor for the names of hospitals at which he or she has medical staff privileges. If the physician holds staff privileges only at a remote hospital, you should inquire why.

If you live in either a rural or inner-city area, you need to be aware that hospitals in these areas may have difficulty in attracting top-quality specialists. While the growth in the number of physicians has greatly increased from one physician for every 641 Americans in 1970 to one for every 420 in 1988, the proportion of physicians in rural and inner-city areas has not risen. It is possible that the less competent doctor who has received disciplinary action or who has lost his or her local hospital staff privileges might opt to apply for staff privileges at a rural or inner-city hospital.

## Eight Symptoms of the Inappropriate Doctor

The quality of the relationship between you and your doctor should initially have nothing to do with trust. Trust is not the issue. You should proceed independently of trust. Your primary goal should be to obtain the quality of medical service that you desire. Focusing on trust will hinder your ability to effectively screen physicians as you search for the right doctor. For example, the patient who develops a blind trust in a doctor on the very first visit may have difficulty objectively evaluating the treatment plan. Build with your doctor a relationship based upon sound questioning, open communications, and mutual expectations of services. Trust will then develop over a period of time.

You probably do not have the "right" doctor if your doctor displays any of the following eight symptoms:

*SYMPTOM 1: Seems to be Dr. "I-Don't-Know"—* You should receive straightforward answers to your questions. If your doctor consistently responds that he or she does not know the answer or that he or she will consult the medical books or other physicians, you either have a very difficult-to-diagnose illness, or the physician is not the foremost authority. In either case, it's time to seek an opinion elsewhere.

*SYMPTOM 2: Causes feelings of avoidance—* Beware of the doctor who does not focus or concentrate on your specific medical problem, such as if your doctor continuously gets off the track, relies too heavily upon staff members, completes an inadequate physical examination, repeatedly cancels clinics, fails to spend adequate time with you, is reluctant to allow second opinions, fails to address your concerns, or appears to be preoccupied with other things. Be wary of the doctor who makes big promises for proposed treatment and downplays the associated risks. This "pie in the sky" approach can lead to unreasonable expectations. Then, if the treatment results are less successful than promised, resentment can occur. The doctor might then try to avoid you or even blame you for the unsatisfactory outcome. Basically, if your intuition is making you feel uncertain about the doctor, even though you cannot pinpoint any specific reasons, trust your instinct. Go to another doctor.

*SYMPTOM 3: Lacks results*—Some indications that your doctor may be stumped are if he or she keeps ordering tests; if your medication is regularly altered slightly; or if you do not see any improvement in your condition. For example, if the doctor appears uncertain of a diagnosis after completing a battery of tests, or makes a vague diagnostic assumption such as stress or some psychosomatic disorder, he or she may have reached a dead end. Insist on going elsewhere for another opinion.

*SYMPTOM 4: Offers a poor prognosis*—If your doctor offers you a poor prognosis, you most likely have a very serious illness, the wrong treatment plan, or the wrong doctor. In any event, it's time to consult other specialists. For example, if the doctor gives you two years to live or states that you will just have to live with your chronic illness, the doctor may not have the necessary skills, or may not even be aware of other treatment options. Even if the prognosis is true, you owe it to yourself to consult other doctors in order to confirm the prognosis or to prevent unnecessary pain or disability.

*SYMPTOM 5: Overprescribes drugs*—Beware of the doctor who prescribes too many drugs to treat your problem (a practice sometimes referred to as *polypharmacy*). An example is an orthopedic specialist who saw a patient for a simple ankle sprain resulting from a worker's compensation injury and who went on to prescribe six different medications ranging from anti-depression medication for his temporary disability, an anti-inflammatory and a cortiosteroid for the ankle, vitamins and minerals for his general health, a medication for his sensitive stomach, a different heart medication (without consulting the patient's cardiologist), and finally, a medication to combat the potential side effects of all the other medications. This doctor also ordered several diagnostic tests consisting of laboratory blood work, X-rays, and an MRI scan.

The doctor did all this on the first visit just because of a single work-related ankle injury. How would the doctor know which medications worked and which did not? What unnecessary risks did this doctor pose to the patient? The patient not only did not need all these medications and tests, but the worker's compensation carrier refused to pay for most of them, deeming them unnecessary and excessive. The worker compensation insurance carrier then sent the patient to another specialist, who prescribed aspirin and an ankle support, which resolved the patient's problem. The message here is: Consult another opinion anytime a doctor wants to do too much too fast, whether it be tests, medications, or surgical treatment.

*SYMPTOM 6: Makes you feel controlled, manipulated, or confused*—The quality of the relationship between you and your doctor should be a reciprocal one built on good communication and mutual expectations. Beware of the doctor who tries to make you dependent on him or her or who attempts to persuade you into treatment. Some doctors' offices are referred to as the "black hole" by the local insurance and medical community because whenever a new patient enters his or her office, the patient seems to remain there forever and is never released from the doctor's care. The doctor makes the patient dependent upon him or her by continually prescribing medications (that need renewals), always finding a new ailment to treat, and requiring frequent (and generally, unnecessary) office visits. A healthy relationship exists if the patient is getting better or is released to another doctor if treatment is not working within a reasonable period of time.

*SYMPTOM 7: Your doctor is not a specialist for your medical problem*—As pointed out in chapter 1, make sure that the doctor is a board-certified specialist or subspecialist for your particular medical problem. Some doctors may claim to be specialists but are either not board-certified, lack training, or lack sufficient experience in your type of disease. In many states a doctor has an unlimited license to practice medicine, which essentially allows him or her to practice in a wide variety of areas. Although hospitals may regulate in which given areas a physician can practice, you still should inquire about the doctor's expertise. Be wary of the doctor who advertises an array of services and implies being a specialist in these areas. The doctor may be driven more by financial market trends than by a special interest and expertise in a given area.

*SYMPTOM 8: Has treated only a few of your type of case*—All other factors considered equal, would you rather be treated by a specialist who treats only one or two of your type of case per year or one who treats several? Common sense tells us that we will most likely obtain a better result with the doctor who treats more cases of a specific type of disease than one who does not. Find a doctor who is not only a specialist or subspecialist in your medical problem but who also devotes his or her primary career to treating your type of problem and regularly treats many of these cases each year. Chapter 5 will cover "Asking the Right Questions" to help you determine the expertise of a doctor.

## How To Know If You Have the Wrong Hospital

Hospitals have gone through several significant changes during the past decade. The changes in the Medicare reimbursement program and escalating health-insurance premiums have caused hospitals to move toward more outpatient care, specialty services, and specialized diagnostic testing. From seventy-seven percent in 1970 to sixty-six percent in 1989, the decrease in the number of full beds in hospitals has mandated that hospitals become more competitive and concerned with their survival. All these changes have an impact on the quality of your care. If you select the right doctor, you will most likely be admitted to the most appropriate hospital. Even so, you still need to be concerned with the fact that differences do exist among hospitals and that the ultimate selection of a doctor might be dependent upon the hospital that he or she uses.

Consider the *ABC News Prime Time Live* segment entitled "Surgical Scorecards" that was broadcast on June 4, 1992. This segment discussed New York State's system of using a scorecard to rank thirty hospitals and 140 heart surgeons who perform bypass surgeries; rankings are based on the number of cases and mortality rates (percentage of deaths). The hospitals' mortality rate for bypass surgeries ranged from less than two percent to almost nine percent. As an example, one hospital performed more than one thousand bypasses a year, with a 3.6 percent mortality rate, as compared with another hospital that performed just over one hundred bypasses, with more than twice the mortality rate. Wide variations also exist among the physicians' mortality rates. At one Manhattan hospital, one surgeon had done 324 bypass surgeries in a two-year period, with one death; another surgeon at the same hospital had done eighty-seven bypasses, with ten deaths. The conclusion of the segment was that quality-care differences among hospitals and physicians exist, that high volume suggests better results, and that patients have a right to know these differences. Pennsylvania, Iowa, and Colorado have also begun systems of rating hospitals and/or physicians. Though several risk factors can affect the validity of these statistics, nevertheless, information like this can be vital in helping you select the right doctor and hospital.

The Health Care Financing Administration (HCFA), which manages the national Medicare program, studies mortality rates for nearly 60,000 hospitals in the country. Its report, entitled *Medicare Hospital Mortality Information*, consists of volumes of books, broken down by states. In compiling the statistical information, several patient-risk factors are considered, such as age, sex, diagnosis, and severity of illness. The mortality rates are categorized under sixteen different diagnostic areas and are compared with a predetermined range of predicted death rates. Even though this information is certainly not a perfect measure of the quality of care of a hospital, it can be very useful to you in assessing the quality of care of hospitals.

You need to recognize that there are a number of situations that can affect the hospital results of being statistically too high or too low. Some of these might include coding differences among hospitals, outright diagnostic coding errors, type of patient population, level of difficult cases treated, and type of hospital services provided (e.g., chronically ill facility vs. acute-care hospital). In fact,

> When properly understood and used, this information can be useful; it can also be very misleading if interpreted incorrectly. The information simply describes one aspect of individual hospital performances—post-admission mortality for Medicare beneficiaries. The information is not necessarily representative of a hospital's total performance in all aspects of patient care . . . Consumers should read the explanations of the uses and limitations of the information, as well as any comments a hospital may have provided.[16]

Though the HCFA mortality report has been met with controversy among the medical community, it can help hospitals to examine and improve the quality of their care and allow the public some measure of comparison among hospitals. The Public Citizen Health Research Group, started by Ralph Nader and headed by Dr. Sidney Wolfe, supports the HCFA study:

> This (HCFA mortality report) allows the public, which includes patients, families, hospital administrators, doctors, insurance officers, and government officials, to openly explore the reasons behind these differences and to work toward reducing the number of preventable deaths. We applaud HCFA for this major public information effort.[17]

However, *U.S. News & World Report* states that "The government's findings are minimally helpful . . . and 68 percent of physicians responded that it is not at all useful, and an additional 17 percent said they do not know what to make of the data."[18]

The HCFA report is available to the public from HCFA, Social Security offices, regional American Association of

Retired Persons (AARP) offices, and some hospitals and libraries. For further information, contact Health Care Financing Administration, Health Standards and Quality Bureau, 2-D-2 Meadows East Building, 6325 Security Blvd., Baltimore, MD 21207 (301-966-1133).

When analyzing a hospital, you need to be concerned not only with mortality rates but also infection rates, patient satisfaction results, quality of operating rooms (e.g., air flow system, operating room procedures, infection-prevention attire, type of equipment), risk-management controls, emergency room coverage, diagnostic laboratory capabilities, intensive care units, and so on. Ask the doctors you are screening about the quality of hospital services as compared with other hospitals. Many doctors and medical personnel will be frank in their comparisons of hospitals, and you can learn a great deal of information to help you make a decision.

You can be assured that the effort to improve the quality of hospital care is continual. Most states now have quality health commissions, and organizations such as JCAHO (Joint Commission on Accreditation of Healthcare Organizations) are developing quality-care indexes and public brochures. To receive a free brochure, send a self-addressed, stamped envelope to "Helping You Choose" Brochures, Customer Service Center, JCAHO, Renaissance Blvd., Oakbrook Terrace, IL 60181.

There are many different types of hospitals—private, nonprofit, acute care, chronically ill, super clinics, specialty clinics, university-affiliated teaching, and so on—all having various characteristics and degrees of expertise. Dr. Herbert Dietrich, in his book, *The Best In Medicine*, suggests that the best hospitals are those that are university-affiliated teaching hospitals. He cites five reasons:

1. The teaching centers have the latest diagnostic tools.
2. They have the trained surgical-medical teams who have worked together many times and know how to handle any situation that may arise from your illness.
3. They have the most experienced surgeons, based on number of patients treated annually.
4. They are academic in motivation, no matter who the patient may be.
5. They receive state and federal grants, which help to offset the costs of patient care.[19]

Because your illness or your unique situation may narrow your hospital choices, talk with your doctors, medical personnel, and organizations to help you to select the right hospital for you. To aid you in your selection, Appendix D lists the best hospitals and clinics across the nation, according to *U.S. News & World Report*. Appendix E lists other sources of hospital surveys.

### Six Characteristics of a Good Patient

Part of the responsibility of obtaining quality care from your doctor rests on you, the patient. Many people are "difficult" patients, which can adversely affect the doctor's relationship with them. Unfortunately, these patients do not realize that their behaviors are hurting their chances of receiving the best health care possible. In fact, doctors and staff cringe at the sight of certain patients who often end up going from doctor to doctor, never realizing that *they* themselves are the problem. To make optimum use of your time with the doctor so that you can obtain the best possible health care, exhibit "good" patient behaviors and avoid being a difficult patient.

*CHARACTERISTIC 1—Have a positive attitude.* Many patients tend to complain openly about anything and everything, to other people in the waiting room, to the office staff, and to the doctor. This type of patient is referred to as "the complainer." The doctor will often react by "tuning out" the complainer, which results in a shorter, unproductive office visit. Complainers not only affect their own health care, but they have an impact on other people who have to listen to them; these people, in turn, can then become stressed and join in the complaining session. While everyone might have legitimate complaints from time to time, vocalize your complaints sparingly and only if essential to your health care.

*CHARACTERISTIC 2—Be honest with your doctor.* You need to tell the doctor precisely the symptoms and pain you have been feeling. Your doctor cannot help you if you do not give him or her all the necessary information that is vital to your care. Do not downplay your symptoms of illness, even if you're embarrassed, afraid of potential tests, or fearful of the potential diagnosis. Patients who exhibit this behavior are called "gatekeepers." An example of a gatekeeper is a person who will regale anyone who will listen with all the pain and symptoms that he has been experiencing, yet during an office visit, he will tell the doctor that he is feeling fine. Gatekeepers resort to this behavior out of an underlying fear of the diagnosis, concern about costly tests, fear of the prognosis, or inconvenience they may impose on others.

*CHARACTERISTIC 3—Communicate effectively.* Listen intently to the doctor and staff. Ask questions and state opinions in a straightforward, respectful manner; avoid condescending or sarcastic behavior. A common and frustrating type of patient for doctors is the "know-it-all." This patient may have some medical experience or is used to being in an authoritative or controlling role and thinks that he or she knows as much as the doctor does. The know-it-all tactlessly questions every decision and can make life difficult for the entire staff. After their visits with a doctor, know-it-alls enjoy bragging to friends and relatives about how much they know about medicine as compared with their doctor. The know-it-alls' behavior quite often results from resistance or denial of the seriousness of their medical condition because they do not feel in control, or because of an inferiority complex.

*CHARACTERISTIC 4—Take responsibility.* If treatment is not progressing as expected, then calmly and confidently do what needs to be done: Talk to the doctor and ask questions and switch doctors if necessary. Do not become obsessed with blaming the doctor. If you disagree or feel uncomfortable with a diagnosis, prognosis, treatment plan, or outcome, remain calm. Do not "blow up" or display anger with the doctor. Your anger will get you nowhere and may cause the doctor to shy away from becoming further involved in your care. Your anger may also carry over to the next doctor, jeopardizing future medical care. For example, Dr. Ben Carson, in his book, *Think Big*, describes a situation in which he referred a mother elsewhere because of her past practice of threats of malpractice lawsuits and her negative, angry attitude. No doctor wants this type of patient, the "blamer"—nothing can be more humiliating or discouraging for a doctor who has done his or her best than to get a frivolous malpractice claim. Assume responsibility for your care and recognize that there are many deterrents to quality health care.

*CHARACTERISTIC 5—Confront your medical problem.* If you have a medical problem, deal with it. Do not indulge in self-pity or accept chronic pain or a health condition just because you think that no one will be able to help you anyway. Difficult patients, termed "negative," tend to view outside influences (insurance companies, hospitals, fate) as having more control than their doctor or themselves in dictating their medical conditions. Negatives have a deep-seated, pessimistic attitude, often based on their beliefs and religious convictions. They generally do not make much effort to try to improve their health condition, because they feel that no one will be able to help them anyway. Avoid a defeatist attitude. Take a positive approach and maintain your hope and optimism even during difficult times.

*CHARACTERISTIC 6—Be organized and knowledgeable.* Take an interest in learning about your medical problem. Become as informed as possible. You will then be able to carry on an intelligent discussion with your doctor and even ask questions about his treatment plan, diagnosis, and prognosis. When you visit a doctor, bring necessary medical records with you and your notes and questions.

In summary, a good patient is responsible, courteous, considerate, and listens to the doctor and staff; intelligently questions decisions; is informed of his or her medical disease; and is supportive of the health-care system. A good patient will have the optimum chance of receiving quality medical care.

# 5

# Networking
# for the Right Doctor

*By now you should have* a fairly thorough understanding of
your particular medical problem and treatment alternatives.
Hopefully, you have started a list of doctors and facilities
throughout the country that deal with your particular
medical problem. You should also have a basic understanding of the inner workings of the medical system. You are
now ready to begin the networking process to find the right
doctor for you.

## Formula A-Z

The networking process of finding the right doctor is not
a sophisticated approach. It is basic common sense. Networking is the process of establishing a communications
exchange among many individuals and institutions. For
example, have you ever thrown a rock into the water and
watched the ripple effect as the waves continue to spread out
farther and farther? Just as a wave multiplies itself in ever-
widening ripples, so will your medical referral network
broaden.

Finding the right doctor is similar to job hunting. It is a
well-planned, systematic approach, requiring strict disci-
pline, patience, good detective skills, record keeping, and
follow-up. One simple networking technique is called

*Referral Network List*

#1.    Name            _____

       Profession      _____

       Phone #         _____

       Referred By     _____

       Comments        _____

                       _____

                       _____

#2.    Name            _____

       Profession      _____

       Phone #         _____

       Referred By     _____

       Comments        _____

                       _____

                       _____

#3.    Name            _____

       Profession      _____

       Phone #         _____

       Referred By     _____

       Comments        _____

                       _____

                       _____

**Figure 5–1. A practical referral network list.**

Formula A-Z. It simply means talking to as many people as you can about your medical problem. Don't be embarrassed to ask an opinion of every person with whom you have contact—your dentist, librarian, appliance serviceperson, and so on. Formula A-Z, therefore, implies that you talk to everyone, from A (anesthetists) to Z (zoologists). Don't underestimate the information and knowledge of other people. Persons from whom you least expect results can often pull through for you. Others might have heard of a doctor or read a clipping from a newspaper that can give you valuable leads.

Utilize all your available sources that you have been gathering, such as surveys, research publications, newspapers, registers of doctors, hospitals, hotline services, associations, and consulting and referral groups. Prepare a referral list by using a form such as the one in Figure 5-1 and list all the potential referral facilities and doctors that you will be calling.

Begin your networking approach by calling the different doctors and facilities on your referral list. You should briefly explain the medical problem, ask who (he or she feels) is the current expert for this type of medical problem, and ask his or her opinion about your case. You will often be given names of other physicians. Take good notes and don't be afraid to ask questions. Mail your medical records promptly if requested. Be aware of self-serving interests and politics and be cautious about ulterior intentions and motives. Most times, however, physicians will be very sincere and generous with their time and information. Remember, though, that physicians are constantly in fear of being sued for malpractice and may be reluctant to comment too much on a specific case without having seen the patient. They may also be reluctant to recommend other physicians whom they do not personally know.

## Asking the Right Questions

Most individuals do not know how to ask the appropriate questions to assess the skills and abilities of a doctor. Their questions are often sketchy and shallow. You must structure your questions to gain the necessary, crucial information about a doctor. Figure 5-2 gives examples of inappropriate questions (i.e., less effective) and appropriate questions (i.e., more effective). The questions are based on a case of a child with a brain tumor.

The purpose of examining the different types of questions in Figure 5-2 is to understand the "art of effective questioning"—to get you thinking about how and why questions are so important as well as to develop your questioning skills so that you get results. Let's explore the meaning behind some of these questions. For example, "If it were your child, what would you do?" is a very common question. Since the parents are overwhelmed with love and compassion for their child, it is understandable that they would ask this question. This question, however, is too emotionally based. Asking a doctor this hypothetical question places him or her in a very difficult position inasmuch as it is difficult to correlate between a surgeon's own child, another child, and his or her surgical skills. Therefore, most surgeons are likely to respond by indicating that they feel comfortable in treating your child. The question "Do you feel confident?" is too abstract. Most doctors tend to have very well-nurtured egos and are confident people. With this question you are actually addressing the doctor's credibility. Questions too vague and general in nature do not get at the intended results—what you want to achieve. Structure your questions so that the answers can be quantifiable. This will allow you to evaluate logically the responses.

If a doctor is evasive in responding to a question, you

| Wrong Questions (Less Effective) | Right Questions (More Effective) |
|---|---|
| • If it were your child, what would you do? | • How many surgeries specifically in resecting Astrocytomas—Grade #1 in the cerebellum, compacted on the brain stem of four-year-old children, have you done? |
| • Do you feel confident? | • Of the surgeries that you have performed like this, were you unable to resect the total tumor, or partially? |
| • Have you done these types of surgeries before? | • Explain to me specifically your approach in removing this tumor and the risks. |
| • How do you think everything will go? | • What are the results that you realistically feel will be achieved—(worst and best)? |
| • Should I have the surgery? | • What if I don't have surgery? What post-operative therapy will be needed? What are other alternatives? |
| • Can you help us decide a treatment plan? | • Is this type of surgery your primary specialty? |
| • Is this the best procedure? | • Is the surgery experimental? |

**Figure 5–2. Examples of wrong (ineffective) and right (effective) questions.**

may need to rephrase or repeat the question. For example, if you ask the doctor how many brain surgeries he or she has performed and the doctor replies, "I have performed hundreds of brain surgeries," you should respond, "Yes, but how many have you performed of this specific type in children?" If the response is, "Only a few, and nobody does too many," you should be skeptical of the doctor's experience and skills.

Be very suspicious of questions that are answered in a roundabout fashion. Look for straight answers, not "wishy-washy" ones. If at all possible, although it may be difficult, talk to people in the medical community about the experience and skills of the various doctors. Doctors form a reputation in both the public and medical community that may not always be the same. For example, there was a surgeon in a small city who had built a good reputation in the public eye because of his well-publicized newspaper articles, fancy office building, and the fact that he was the local university's sports physician. However, many of the front-line medical practitioners—surgical technicians, operating room nurses, floor nurses, physical therapists, and doctor assistants—knew differently. They all knew that he was sloppy in the operating room, not conscientious, rough in surgery, and often inattentive with post-operative medical care. Don't overlook the opinions of the medical staff. Though you may not always get a true opinion from these medical people since they may work with a doctor, it is surprising how these people can indirectly steer you in the right direction.

When talking to the doctor, think of yourself as a consultant or private investigator. Remember to be assertive but polite. Do not tolerate highly complicated medical terms and technical jargon. You are the consumer, not the doctor. Don't be afraid to ask about the doctor's professional

## Other Helpful Questions

- How much will the treatment cost?
- What is your philosophy towards therapy?
- Where will treatment take place—in your office or a hospital?
- Is the procedure inpatient or outpatient?
- What are the specific risks?
- Who will be assisting you on the case?
- How long will treatment/surgery take?
- What special insurance requirements are necessary?
- What is the length of recovery?
- What is the mortality rate and other possible complications?
- What special care needs to be done after treatment?
- How will I benefit from this surgery or treatment?
- Are you aware of any other treatments or different approaches for this problem?
- Please tell me names of some other skilled experts.
- Please tell me names of patients who have had this procedure.
- How are the facilities and patient care at the hospital?
- Has the hospital where you will be doing the procedure been experienced in handling this type of procedure?
- What will be the type of medication or special therapy requirements?
- What should I look for after surgery that would indicate a problem?
- What are some possible side-effects?
- Do the benefits outweigh the risks?
- What are the chances of recurrence? Are there long-term risks?
- What will happen if we don't do surgery?

## Telephone Networking Worksheet

Doctor's Name _____ Date _____

Specialty _____ Institution _____

Objective of Call        (For Example: to obtain an opinion)

Step 1 Introduction      Introduce yourself

Step 2 Referral          State who referred you

Step 3 Case Problem      Briefly state case (e.g., four-year-
old child with astrocytoma grade #1 in cerebellum with
residual tumor.) Operated on (date) by Dr. (name) only small
portion removed. Describe current symptoms.

Step 4 Opinion           Ask Doctor's opinion.

_____

_____

Step 5 Record Comments   _____

_____

_____

Step 6 Next Step         Write down next step.

_____

_____

Step 7 Closing           Summarize discussion. Thank Doctor.

_____

_____

**Documentation**. Summarize your discussion, gut feelings, specific concerns, positives and negatives, etc.

_____

_____

_____

_____

**Figure 5–3. Utilizing a Telephone Networking Worksheet.**

background, training, and how much experience he or she has had with your specific disease. Ask how many cases of this specific disease the doctor has treated and use this number as a comparison with other doctors. Perhaps you might ask for names of other patients whom the doctor has treated. While you may only receive names of satisfied customers, you can surprisingly still learn much from them. Talk to other patients in the waiting room or to medical professionals in the office.

## Telephone Prospecting

The telephone is a quick, efficient way to gain prospects. If you cannot reach the doctor, give your telephone number and ask that your call be returned. If the doctor doesn't call you back, don't hesitate to call again. Recognize that doctors are busy and have family lives, too. If you get desperate, you can always try calling the doctor at home, particularly in serious situations. It helps to use a telephone worksheet when initiating your calls, such as the one shown in Figure 5-3.

At times it may be difficult to reach a doctor by phone. You may need a "hook" to get you through. In our case, we were fortunate that Dan could use his Ph.D. degree to introduce himself as "Dr. Tomal," which would generally give him direct contact. However, once when he was connected to a prestigious physician, the physician's first comment to Dan was, "What type of M.D. are you?" Dan replied, "I'm not an M.D. I have a Ph.D., and I'm just a desperate parent trying to save my child's life from a brain tumor." With that, the physician replied, "Well, how can I help you?"

Most people do not have a "Dr." in front of their name, so one way to access a doctor by phone is to start with the medical office staff. Talk to the receptionist and other office personnel; they will often be helpful and compassionate and make special provisions to get you through to the doctor. Ask for the office manager and tell him or her that you have good health insurance; you may then be more readily connected with the doctor. Remember that the doctor's practice is a business. Not all medical businesses want to take on a very difficult, time-consuming, legally risky medical case, especially if they will be poorly paid, or not paid at all. However, don't let the fact that you have poor health insurance, an unsettled accident case, or no insurance at all dampen your enthusiasm when your health, or that of a family member, is at stake. Many doctors and hospitals will take on no-pay/high-risk cases purely for philanthropic reasons.

Another excellent way to gain information and access to the doctor is through his or her right-hand assistant. Almost all doctors have an assistant, such as a charge nurse, business manager, administrative manager, or physician assistant, who is the backbone behind the doctor's practice. This assistant is generally very skilled and knowledgeable about the specific diseases and treatment procedures. You can gain an incredible amount of information from this person. The assistant often serves as a screen and go-between for the doctor as well as handles much of his or her written communication and business. The assistant can often effectively explain information to you more clearly than the doctor will and can also provide you with resources and videotapes. Also, ask the assistant what time is best to reach the doctor. Find out when the doctor has clinic, office hours, or makes rounds. Some doctors can be reached during clinic hours, between patients. You may be placed on hold, but at least you'll eventually get through. Some doctors may refuse calls during clinic hours, so you might try paging the doctor during his or her hospital rounds. For some doctors, you

```
Date

Doctor's Name
Doctor's Address

Dear Doctor:

I would like to ask your opinion about my four-year-old
boy, Jonathan, who has a brain tumor.

Last November, Jonathan, a healthy child, started
having intermittent headaches and some vomiting. A CAT
scan showed a cerebellar tumor just to the left of the
midline. In December he was operated on by a local
neurosurgeon. The surgeon wasn't able to remove the
entire tumor since a fair amount had impacted on the
brain stem. The pathology report indicated the tumor
was an astrocytoma grade #1.

A CAT scan taken a month after the surgery shows a
significant amount of residual tumor. The surgeon
recommends waiting and not reoperating until technology
advances; other surgeons have recommended either
radiation or reoperating.

Jonathan presently is getting worse with increasing
episodes of headaches, which cause him to be bedridden
up to a few hours per day. His coordination at times is
being affected, with difficulty walking straight; and
he often tilts his head to one side.

We look forward to hearing from you and can be reached
at the address or telephone number below. Also, if you
desire, we can send you a copy of his CAT scans and
pathology slide.

Sincerely,


Your Name

Your Address
Telephone Number

cc: Neurosurgeon
    Pediatrician
```

**Figure 5–4. A Sample opinion letter**

might try anticipating when the doctor is traveling between the office and hospital, since many of them have car phones and can easily talk to you.

## Correspondence

In addition to using the telephone, you may need to write letters to doctors or medical institutions, explaining your medical problem. State the purpose of your letter up front. Present the problem; provide a brief background on the case; and give the name of your family physician, the doctor who diagnosed the problem, and the person who referred you to him or her. If necessary, include the supporting information, such as doctors' reports, pathology, slides, or copies of X-rays. Conclude your letter by making a bid for action, such as "Please call me." Figure 5-4 presents a sample letter.

Some key points in writing letters include:

1. State the purpose of your letter up front.

2. Empathize with the recipient of the letter. Put yourself in his or her shoes. This will help you structure the content of the letter.

3. Be as specific as possible; try to give all the facts and details. For example, rather than just stating that you have a cancer, state the specific type.

4. Organize the information in chronological order, describing when symptoms were first experienced, past treatments, other opinions, and present condition.

5. Try to get a referral to a specialist from your primary-care physician. Ask that he or she send a letter as well.

## Monitoring Your Progress

Be patient during your search and *don't give up on God*. It is easy to become depressed and to give up hope, but you

| DOCTOR'S NAME | COMMENTS: |
|---|---|
| 1. *Pediatric Neurosurgeon* | *Recommendation*: Operate soon. |
| Date _____ | (Summarize the doctor's |
| Institution _____ | comments.) |
| Address _____ | |
| Telephone _____ | |
| 2. *Neurosurgeon* | *Recommendation*: Do radiation, not surgery. |
| Date _____ | (Summarize the doctor's |
| Institution _____ | comments.) |
| Address _____ | |
| Telephone _____ | |
| 3. *Neurosurgeon* | *Recommendation*: Wait; do not operate yet. |
| Date _____ | (Summarize the doctor's |
| Institution _____ | comments.) |
| Address _____ | |
| Telephone _____ | |
| 4. *Brain-Tumor Researcher* | *Recommendation*: Consider surgery and radiation combination. |
| Date _____ | (Summarize the doctor's |
| Institution _____ | comments.) |
| Address _____ | |
| Telephone _____ | |
| 5. *Oncologist* | *Recommendation*: Consider surgery vs. chemotherapy or radiation. |
| Date _____ | (Summarize the doctor's |
| Institution _____ | comments.) |
| Address _____ | |
| Telephone _____ | |

**Figure 5–5. Example of monitoring the networking process, using a sample hypothetical case of a child with a brain tumor.**

must keep your faith and remember that God has his own timetable.

As you proceed with your discussions with doctors, you must effectively monitor your search campaign. Be detailed in recording your comments. It is helpful to type your information, since you will most likely need to send it to others for their review and opinions. Using a hypothetical situation of a child with a brain tumor, Figure 5-5 presents an example of how you can record and monitor your progress.

## Dealing with Mixed Opinions

As you can see from the hypothetical situation (Figure 5-5), doctors had varying opinions: (a) wait; (b) radiate; (c) operate soon; (d) use a combination of surgery and radiation. A variety of opinions is not unusual, especially when the doctors have various specialties and subspecialties. For example, if you talk only to doctors who specialize in radiation treatment, you are apt to receive many opinions to treat the illness with radiation. It is important, therefore, that you solicit opinions from different subspecialists.

Doctors make their opinions based upon their own personal experiences, skills, knowledge, specialty (or sub-specialty), intuition, and posture (conservative or more aggressive). With this in mind, there are bound to be mixed opinions from doctors. But remember, specialists who feel very confident about their opinions will commonly back them up with facts and personal experience.

## As Simple as A, B, C

As you network, you will find the process has three phases, making networking as easy as A, B, C (see Figure 5-6).

*Phase A*—As you begin your search, you will start

developing a short list of names of potential doctors (Figure 5-1). As you continue your search, the list of names of doctors will expand. Always try to talk directly to the doctors on your list about your medical problem.

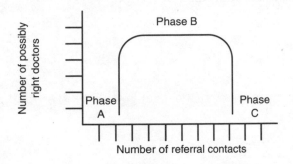

**Figure 5–6**

*Phase B*—In Phase B, as your list continues to grow, it will reach a peak (large list of names). At this point, you should begin to eliminate those doctors who you feel are not the right doctors for your problem. Eliminating certain doctors will be based on responses to your questions, opinions by other doctors, and "gut" reactions.

*Phase C*—As the number of names on the list begins to decrease, the potentially "right" doctors begin to emerge. As you query these top doctors through proper questioning techniques and ask other doctors their opinions of these few top doctors, this process will eventually bring to the surface three to five top doctors to whom you should direct your attention. At this point, make sure that all these top doctors have all the necessary medical information, such as CAT scans, pathology reports, and so on. If possible, schedule an appointment with these top few doctors, but only after they have examined all the information and given you their initial opinion. If a personal appointment is not feasible, you should at least have a very in-depth telephone discussion directly with the doctor. However, you should do your best to schedule an examination with each of these doctors before making your final selection.

# 6

# Selecting the Right Doctor

## Making the Final Decision

*So, what do you do with* your mixed opinions? Now that you have gathered all this information, how do you sort through all of it to actually make a decision about the best doctor, the best treatment plan, or the best medical facility? John Dewey said, "A well-defined problem is half solved." Therefore, by thoroughly examining a medical problem yourself, you will be in a better position to decide upon the proper treatment and doctor. Let's explore some basic principles and strategies.

Once you have completed your search campaign and have collected all the vital information on the doctors and medical treatment, it is time for careful analysis. Essentially, the art of problem solving and decision making involves gathering all available information and logically sorting through it, weighing both the advantages and disadvantages, and then making a decision. As you begin to analyze all the data you have accumulated, keep in mind the following pitfalls to avoid:

1. *Administering treatment before you have an accurate diagnosis*—As we discussed in chapter 1, an accurate diagnosis is a critical first step. For example, you may take aspirin for a headache rather than have the cause diagnosed. Continuing to take aspirin to treat the symptom rather than finding the cause is only postponing the problem, which may

evolve into a more serious problem. If you have a medical problem, don't settle for continued treatment of the symptom. Continue to seek multiple specialists' (or subspecialists') opinions, preferably starting at one large facility. Although this will take time and money, it is the best start as opposed to going to several facilities.

Chapter 2 discussed the concept that a subspecialist may tend to look at a medical condition from the standpoint of his or her personal experience and background. Much too often in medical practice, a particular problem is treated prematurely, based upon a hasty diagnosis and past experience. Realize that quickness in making a diagnosis and decision for treatment can be risky. The doctor could totally miss the medical point at issue that is actually causing the majority of the problems.

2. *Diagnosing a condition when there is none*—As frightful as it sounds, there are reported cases of diagnosing and treating patients for conditions that do not exist, especially in the case of psychosomatic illnesses. Be a wise health consumer and be on guard for non-existent conditions.

3. *Failure to diagnose a disease*—Doctors are limited in their ability and can also make mistakes. The failure to diagnose a disease is not uncommon. For example, breast cancer is a commonly missed disease. The importance of diagnosing it early can make the difference between life and death. Doctors miss this condition for a number of reasons, such as hasty clinical examination, inaccurate mammogram technique, and poor radiological reading. Some physicians take a wait-and-see position when unconvinced of the condition. Use your own feelings, common sense, and spiritual direction. You may be your best health clinician regarding your own body. If you sense that something is wrong and you are not satisfied with your doctor, continue your search.

4. *Making false comparisons*—For example, if you select a doctor for treatment of skin cancer because of his excellent reputation in treating lung cancer, you may not be making the right decision. While the specialist may be an expert in treating one type of cancer, he or she may not be an expert in treating another. Likewise, if a medical facility has an excellent reputation in a given area, this does not mean that its personnel are experts in all areas. Similarly, doctors can make a false diagnosis of a condition and mistake one type of disease for another.

5. *Avoiding the decision*—Avoiding making a decision and not facing up to the problem for fear of the diagnosis, treatment, or effects of treatment can only make the problem worse. Simply giving up your health problem to God and failing to actively listen to him will not solve the problem. It is human nature to avoid negative aspects in life; humans have a tendency to repress negative experiences. In some cases, it may be senseless to prolong treatment any longer if no effective treatment is available.

## Basic Steps for Problem Solving and Decision Making

Let's now consider a process to use in problem solving and decision making. *Problem solving* is defined as the process of troubleshooting and identifying the cause(s) of a medical problem. *Decision making* is the process of selecting the right treatment and doctor. Figure 6-1 presents seven basic steps in problem solving and decision making.

Let's examine these steps in more detail, using the hypothetical situation in Figure 5-5.

1. *Diagnosing the problem*—The first step is to be very clear in identifying the true *cause* of the problem, not the symptom. For example, in the case of a child's brain tumor, the headaches are the symptom, and the tumor of astrocy-

toma in the cerebellum is the cause. It is important in diagnosing the problem to get a very detailed and accurate description of the cause or multiple causes for your medical condition.

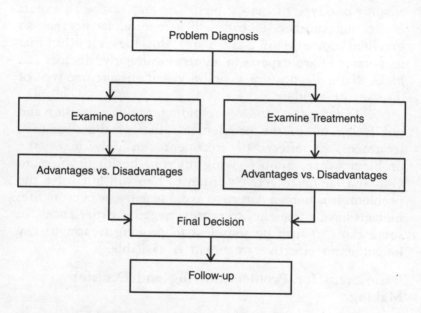

1.  Diagnosing the problem
2.  Examining all possible doctors and facilities
3.  Examining all proposed treatment plans
4.  Understanding fully each treatment plan outlined by each doctor
5.  Weighing the advantages and disadvantages
6.  Making a final decision
7.  Follow-up and evaluation (monitoring progress, physical therapy, postoperative care, etc.)

**Figure 6–1. Seven basic steps in problem solving and decision making**

2. *Examining all possible doctors or facilities as alternatives*—List all the doctors and facilities and analyze all the available facts and information. Opinions supported by numbers of cases and actual results, research, and experience are much more valuable than unsubstantiated words.

3. *Examining all proposed treatments*—In analyzing all possible alternatives, consider the facts of the actual treatment for your specific type of case and not speculations. To help understand the alternative treatments, separate the "what is" from the "what is not." The treatment may be good for some tumors, for example, but not for your specific type. Also avoid emotional reasoning at this stage. Strengthen your creative thinking by suspending judgments on ideas or treatments that are different and don't be afraid to take a chance. Don't let your fear prevent you from choosing a specific treatment as long as you have explored all the possible choices and understand all the possible risks and side effects.

It is important to separate the treatment from the doctor. You may feel extremely comfortable with a specific doctor, yet his or her skill or treatment plan may not be the best for your particular problem. You may first want to consider the alternative treatments. For example, the treatments in the hypothetical example are as follows:

A. Do nothing; wait until technology advances.

B. Do surgery soon.

C. Do radiation.

D. Do chemotherapy.

E. Do a combination of surgery and radiation.

F. Continue to see other doctors.

4. *Understanding*—You should next clarify your situation by fully understanding each of the treatments and skills of the doctors. For example, although radiation is an

alternative in the hypothetical situation, it may produce possible long-term development problems.

The use of synergism can be a powerful strategy in clarifying your information and making an intelligent decision. Synergism suggests that groups make better decisions than single individuals make. Solicit the help of friends and relatives to help you think through the information so that you can make the best decision. This synergistic approach is also a key advantage in large medical facilities, where a team of specialists can discuss the difficult cases.

5. *Weighing the advantages and disadvantages*—Weighing the advantages and disadvantages can be frustrating and difficult, especially in life-threatening situations. The best approach is to actually write down on paper each treatment and doctor, listing the advantages and then the disadvantages. Place a value or degree on the importance of each one. There will always be a gray area, so don't let this hinder your decision.

6. *Make a final decision*—After examining the advantages and disadvantages, you should pray to God for his guidance and then select the best treatment and doctor. It can sometimes be difficult to make a final selection. In some cases you might confer with persons other than your close friends or relatives. These individuals can give their unbiased opinions and often think more clearly because they are not emotionally involved. Furthermore, when two doctors are very capable and qualified and seem equal in all respects, you may want to go to the one with whom you feel more comfortable, the one who's located more conveniently, or the one affiliated with the better medical institution and supporting medical staff. Keep in mind that once you have selected the best doctor, don't disregard selection of the best supporting medical staff members. These individuals might include the anesthesiologist, operating physician assistant,

rehabilitative specialist, follow-up specialist, physical therapist, and so on. For example, the anesthesiologist is often unknown and taken for granted by the patient. Authors Cohan, Primm, and Jude emphasize this point in their book, *A Patient's Guide to Heart Surgery*[20]:

> The anesthesiologist is the most critical person on the surgery team, yet traditionally this is one area where patients are given no choice . . . as surgeons and operating room nurses often confide, if they were patients, they would be sure to choose a specific one or two anesthesiologists . . .

You should be aware that many hospitals use nurse anesthetists instead of anesthesiologists who are medical doctors. Since the nurse anesthetist is often an employee of the hospital, the hospital can bill out for the anesthesiology services. Although many nurse anesthetists are very good, you may feel more comfortable with an anesthesiologist. When selecting supporting medical staff members, talk to your specialist and other medical personnel.

7. *Follow-up evaluation*—Remember that every treatment should be followed up with periodic examinations. In some cases the treatment may need to be followed with special care, medication, or therapy. You should determine your follow-up with your doctor and select the best follow-up medical staff as well.

Once you have made your decision, accept the responsibility for it and face it with a positive attitude. Recognize that it was the best alternative based upon well-informed research. Accept the results of the treatment as well but be flexible should you need to make additional decisions or to seek other care.

# 7

# Victory Is with God —You Always Win

*Now that you have made a decision* for treatment, you will undoubtedly experience a great deal of stress and varied emotions, especially if surgery is involved. These emotions are often very similar to other life traumas, such as a sudden loss of a job, a car accident, physical disability, or a terminal illness.

A trauma, or life crisis, always initiates a personal threat and change. For centuries the Chinese have known the relationship between crisis and change. The Chinese term for crisis (*wei-ji*) represents the words "danger" and "opportunities." At the onset of a crisis, you will have an extremely hard time believing that in the end, you may be "more, because of it." It is indeed amazing how persons who experience life crises gain wisdom. They often redefine and set new priorities in life and develop a more mature outlook. The value of people and the importance of love, growth, and happiness often take higher meaning than life's small inconveniences and disruptions.

## Stages of Trauma

Research suggests that when people experience a trauma, they normally move through a series of emotional reactions. Some of these emotions include shock, fear, blaming, bargaining, self-pity, resignation, and action. We found ourselves going through these same stages as we dealt with Jonathan's brain tumor.

The initial state of *shock* is common for most people. The shock of discovering the crisis produces a numbness, especially when it is totally unexpected. People will fight the situation, perhaps lie outright, or reject it and appear to be in a daze. A common example of this feeling was vividly experienced and witnessed by millions of people the day John F. Kennedy was shot. People were seen to stand in disbelief. Still today, most people can recall exactly what they were doing when they learned of this tragic event. Nevertheless, in the short run, this denial and disbelief can be healthy because it helps people cope with the initial crisis and allows them to regroup and then face the shocking event.

This first stage often quickly changes to the emotion of *fear*. People panic as they have difficulty accepting the crisis. They become fearful of the unknown and isolation. Thoughts of the worst possible scenario may come, and feelings of desperation and uncertainty may emerge. Direct this fear to God and ask for his comfort and strength.

The *blaming* emotion is generally experienced when denial can no longer be maintained. This emotion can transpose into anger because of the feelings of helplessness. Statements such as, "Why didn't you take him to the doctor earlier?" or "Why me?" or "Why is God punishing me?" are common. The ripping away of security and the intense feelings of vulnerability may be manifested in fits of rage and sometimes violent reaction. Besides anger, the feelings of self-pity, envy, and resentment can occur. A comment such as "Why didn't this happen to someone else?" or outright derogatory remarks toward people who do not have the same problem are common. Examples of this type of expression can be seen in hospitals, where parents spend time in the waiting room while their children are being treated. Parents resent and vocalize the fact that their child will suffer a physical disability while others will not. Parents might also displace their anger toward the doctor, staff, minister, rabbi, or God.

Another stage involves *bargaining*. In this period, people may panic and look toward other options to avoid or postpone the inevitable. For example, people might propose alternatives to the doctor. They might attempt to make a deal with God, such as recommitment of their faith or faithful service in exchange for healing (i.e., something for something). Often in this stage, people may experience severe grief and remorse and may blame themselves.

The stage of *self-pity* is almost inevitable. A person's behavior, such as sleeping, eating, or communication patterns, may radically change. A person also may develop a low self-esteem, a feeling of helplessness, and depression. Attempts to encourage people at this stage are generally met with futility. People take varying degrees of time to overcome this feeling and work through this emotion. The reality of the medical condition is often too much to bear. At times, an event of confrontation with another person can trigger the person out of this stage. Continue to pray for strength, courage, direction, and healing.

During the *resignation* stage, hope, encouragement, and degrees of optimism emerge. People resign themselves to the facts and develop a sense of ownership about their condition, even though they still may experience fear and anxiety. Their energy level increases as they accept their condition and become determined to make the best of it. There is trust and closeness with God. In this stage, thinking becomes clearer and focus is on the future.

The last stage is that of *action*. This stage often includes rebuilding, developing courses of action, setting goals, or coping with the situation. A typical expression is "Well, if this is the will of God, I need to glorify him and make the best of it." New opportunities develop, as you regain a more positive outlook on life. God opens up opportunities that were not there before. The chance to help other people with similar medical conditions as well as opportunities for witness are realized. This is the stage to take charge and put your plan into action.

## Managing Your Stress

In addition to experiencing many stages of emotions, you will also encounter a great deal of stress. How does stress affect us? There are three sources of stress—physical, mental, and emotional. Physical stress can be exhaustion from too much physical work or activity, such as going through rehabilitation, or physically caring for a patient. Mental stress comes from mental exhaustion, such as learning about medical problems and making decisions about medical care, finances, and logistical arrangements. Emotional stress results from the overuse of our emotions, such as in dealing with an accident, disease, awaiting treatment, or a medical emergency. During a crisis you will experience great emotional stress, which you might be able to reduce by physical exercise. Or, if you have had too much physical stress, you can relax and read a book in order to reduce stress. Unfortunately, though, some life-threatening illnesses produce all three stress sources at one time.

Our body's reaction to stress can be compared to waking up in the morning. Our alarm clock sends a signal to wake up; when the alarm clock sounds, we shut it off. In our autonomic nervous system, our internal alarm clock turns our body on and alerts us to something we need to be concerned about; then we need to allow our body to return to a normal condition. An example is if we see flashing police-car lights in the rear-view mirror while driving. Seeing these flashing lights activates our alarm system, which results in increased heart rate, and so forth. Afterward, our body takes over, and we soon return to our normal condition. It is important when dealing with turbulent life situations to be able to recognize and understand how our body operates, to be alerted to the crisis, and to shut our internal alarm system off in order to effectively manage the situation.

Stress itself can be good or bad. Many of the same reactions in our bodies are produced by bad stress (negative stress) or good stress (positive stress). For example, positive stress could be getting married or preparing yourself for a sports event. Positive stress can result in higher productivity, motivation, and success. On the other hand, negative stress, such as witnessing an accident, dealing with illness, or coping with the loss of a loved one, can result in mistakes, nervousness, fatigue, or sickness.

Your attitude plays an important part in whether you view the stress as good or bad and how you deal with the emotional event. You need to trust God during this difficult period. You must face up to the emotional event and try to deal with it with a positive attitude and put your energies into constructive use. For example, if you are faced with a medical illness, rather than dwelling upon the ailment and visualizing all the negative results that could occur, you can channel your efforts into a positive approach. Divert your energies into understanding the problem, exploring possible alternatives, and selecting the right doctor and treatment. This positive approach and use of productive time will be valuable in solving your illness and reducing your stress.

You can manage your stress in several ways:

1. *"Self-talk"*—People have a tendency to talk to them-

selves, especially during stressful periods. This self-talk can be either positive or negative. If you dwell on the negative, you manifest unreasonable expectations and produce even more stress. It is not healthy to focus on a life-threatening illness with the attitude that it will be fatal. Concentrate on the disease with *positive* thinking. Focus on the healing miracle and the promise of treatment. Talk to yourself positively by looking at the pluses and minuses and dealing with them logically. To eliminate negative self-talk, picture a large, red STOP sign and say to yourself—Stop!—to turn off your negative thinking.

2. *Prayer and spiritual strength*—Trust and seek help from God. Build your spiritual strength. Inner strength, direction, and healing from God are important spiritual forces in overcoming difficulties. The peace and tranquility received from God can enable you to reduce your stress and deal with the emotional event. Put the problem in the hands of God. Ask for his mercy and healing power. God will help you through this difficult period.

3. *Positive thoughts*—Whether an event is real or not, the same reactions can occur in your body. For example, when you have a nightmare, you experience the same emotions that you would if you were facing the real event. How often have you walked alone at night and imagined that someone was following you? These feelings are real and are very stressful. Think pleasant thoughts to help you to reduce your stress and aid your recovery. Create a positive mental thought and expectation, such as getting well, or the healing of your body. As you visualize these positive events, your positive attitude can bolster your immune system. Your behavior begins to follow, which, in reality, aids your treatment as you feel less stress.

4. *Self-imposed traps*—Sometimes your greatest enemy can be yourself (i.e., your attitude toward the crisis). You

might impose undue constraints upon yourself. For example, if you've ever been to a circus, you might have noticed that large elephants are often tied by a rope to a small stake. With minimal effort, the elephant could tear away from the pole, but it doesn't. Ever since it was a baby elephant, it has been tied to the pole and conditioned to think that it cannot get away. This conditioning becomes a "self-fulfilling prophecy." What you expect is what you get. If you don't expect much, you don't get much. Eliminate these self-imposed traps that handicap you. Build your confidence and positive expectations.

5. *Build supportive and social relationships*—Talk with other people who have similar problems. This can be very therapeutic during times of emotional crisis. For this reason, hospital waiting rooms can be a very important place to gather. People with mutual concerns can give each other support by listening, caring, ventilating feelings, and giving emotional support. Joining an association that is connected with your medical problem can help since these organizations generally have support groups.

6. *Reconsider the "whole situation"*—When faced with a crisis, rather than dwelling upon the negative aspects, think of the problem in terms of the whole situation. In other words, instead of pouting and sitting around stating, "Ain't it awful?"—look at the problem in terms of how it fits in with your entire life. For example, suppose that you have had an accident and are now handicapped. Rather than dwell upon the specific handicap, look at the entire family unit and be thankful for the health of the other family members or the fact that you are living and productive versus focusing only on the handicap. This "reconsidering process" can help put things in perspective.

7. *Distorted thinking*—You might have a tendency to distort things in times of crisis. You may overgeneralize an

event or see problems as all black-and-white. This can develop into a self-defeatist attitude and produce more stress. Jumping to conclusions or overemotionalizing can interfere with sound decision making. Don't associate every turn of events as more bad news. Separate the good from the bad.

8. *The positive element*—Life has much in common with electricity, wherein positive and negative electrons are essential for energy. We, too, have the "positives" and the "negatives" in life. Sometimes you can have a greater appreciation for the positive things in life through your negative experiences. Therefore, when you encounter a negative experience, deal with it positively, relative to your whole life, and try to find some benefit as a result of the crisis. For example, you might say, "It has been a learning experience," or "We have grown from it and can now help others."

9. *Maintain your health*—It is very easy to disregard your health during the period of a medical problem. The importance of taking vitamins, eating well, getting enough rest and sleep, exercising, and avoiding substance abuse can significantly help to reduce your stress. Though it is sometimes difficult to do, you should encourage yourself to maintain good health practices even during times of trauma.

10. *Fearing the problem*—Sometimes the fear of the problem can be worse than the problem itself. For example, if you are shaking or perspiring because you are nervous about surgery, rather than fight the fear, you can do the opposite—stop resisting it. In other words, instead of "fighting it," accept it. Perceive how nervous you can get, how much you can perspire. This, in turn, may reduce or stop the nervousness or perspiring, since it is often your resistance that is causing the stress rather than the surgery

itself. Accepting stress can help calm you during difficult periods.

11. *Tension relaxers*—Many different quick relaxers can help relieve tension, such as massaging your forehead and back of neck, stretching your muscles, or taking a series of deep breaths. Your spouse or a friend might rub your shoulders and neck. Stretching your muscles will help reduce tension.

12. *Objectivity vs. personalization*—How effectively you deal with stress can be rooted in how you view the event. Some people have a tendency to personalize and internally absorb the medical problem, especially someone else's. Many doctors and nurses, however, in order to give the best care and service to their patients, remove themselves personally from the stressful situation in order to be most effective.

When facing a stressful event, rather than "taking in" everything and emotionally absorbing the event, you might try to externalize it by looking at it from a more objective viewpoint.

13. *Meditation and relaxation*—Self-directed meditation can help reduce your stress. Find a quiet spot and remove all extraneous outside thoughts from entering your mind.

Focus only on God, a pleasant thought, or a word or number. Meditating for just a few minutes per day can be very helpful in coping with your crisis.

14. *Putting things in perspective*—There are some things you can control in life and other things that you cannot control. Try to think of people who are much worse off than you—either medically, financially, emotionally, and so on. Be thankful that you don't have their problems. There are always people worse off than you.

15. *Burnout vs. cop-out*—You can confuse burnout with cop-out. Generally, burnout is experienced when you are

physically, emotionally, or mentally exhausted. Cop-out, on the other hand, is an excuse for not giving one hundred percent. You might, when faced with trauma, use the trauma itself as an excuse for not dealing with the situation (or with life in general). In other words, rather than take a positive approach in dealing with the stressful situation, you avoid it. Your behavior is really an excuse for your dysfunctional attitude. You must ask yourself if you are experiencing burnout or cop-out—and distinguish between the two.

16. *Read helpful books*—Read books on how to cope with stress, books on how other people or parents have dealt with severe medical problems or other life crises. An exceptionally good book that helps put life's events and crises in proper perspective is *When Bad Things Happen to Good People* by Harold Kushner; another book is *Where is God When It Hurts?* by Philip Yancey.

## Helping Family Members Cope

One of the most stressful periods in your life is the tension-filled time prior to treatment (e.g., surgery). This is difficult not only for you but for your family members as well. The pressures of whether you are making the right decisions, the anticipation of the results of the treatment, and the feelings of anxiety can be overwhelming. Here are some ideas and tips that can help you and your family members cope with treatment:

1. *Communication*—Talking to someone can be extremely therapeutic. If you bottle up your feelings and emotions, you need to ventilate them. Don't be afraid to say what you are feeling. This can be a time to develop a real intimacy with your family, relatives, and close friends. Although you might find it difficult to talk to people you don't know well (clergy, nurses, social workers), they are genuinely interested in helping you. The waiting room can

also be an excellent place to share mutual support and reinforce each other. Talking with others who have similar problems is worthwhile. However, talking too much can become counterproductive and might cause you to dwell too much on the problem and not on the solution.

2. *Reflection or restatement*—If you are not the patient, the use of reflection or restatement can be a useful technique in counseling a family member. This technique simply means that you restate exactly what the person said. This helps to clarify the meaning and encourages them to talk more. For example, if a patient or family member says, "I'm worried," you might simply respond, "I'm sure you are" and then be silent. Most likely, the person will continue to talk and to clarify what he means. Also, acknowledge that you are listening, by comments such as, "Go on," "I see," or "I understand."

When you meet a patient or family member and don't know what to say, the best way to start is to ask, "How do you feel?" This allows you to pay attention to their feelings and emotions. For example, a person who had an illness was visited by friends who approached him with extreme anxiety and sorrow. Much to their surprise, they found him to be cheerful. Although he had encountered a tragic illness, he was on the road of slow recovery. Therefore, he was joyful because he was alive and recovering. Conversely, the friends viewed the situation as traumatic and didn't understand his attitude and behavior. When you deal with patients, it is important to ask them how they feel and then respond to them positively, rather than to tell them how you feel. If they are cheerful, respond to them likewise (i.e., reflection). Vice versa, if they feel depressed, comfort them.

3. *Prayer*—The comfort and spiritual strength obtained through prayer can be very healthy for your soul and give you peace of mind. Do not be afraid or embarrassed to pray

with others. Moreover, don't hesitate to ask and to pray for what you feel that you really need. Pray for healing, comfort, direction, and strength.

4. *Activities*—Sometimes it can be helpful if you can gather many books or resources on the illness and read them. This will help to get your mind off the treatment and allow you to become more knowledgeable. Or, during surgery, get out of the hospital and take a walk; focus your mind on other things for a short time.

5. *Be realistic*—Although it is important to be optimistic in dealing with treatment, it is also important to be realistic. For example, don't make such comments as, "Everything will be all right," or "Don't worry; everything is going to be just fine." Although in the end things might very well turn out to be fine, it is difficult for a patient to deal with these statements since they are not based on the facts. The best way to deal with the situation is to deal with it realistically, knowing the risks. Developing false expectations can make it more difficult to emotionally cope later.

## Tips for a Successful Recovery

The mind, body, and soul—three parts of the whole—are equally crucial to your recovery. There are countless stories of people who had illnesses and have physically recovered, but their mind (attitude) did not; eventually these people became destitute, or even died. The mysteries of healing still baffle the greatest minds today. There are remarkable stories of people who were considered terminal but through their determination exceeded the doctors' wildest expectations. Develop a positive attitude, nurture your soul through prayer, and strengthen your body through exercise and good health.

Your recovery may have ups and down. At times you may feel that you are making significant progress and then subsequently you will experience a setback. Have elasticity and bounce back. You should also set short-term and long-term goals for your recovery but do not put specific time frames on them. Physical recovery, unlike goals in the business world, cannot have absolute time frames. Everyone's body recovers at a different rate. In the case of people who have had exactly the same surgeries, it is indeed amazing how some people encounter different problems and recover at a different rate. Much like the flowers of a garden, all will bloom in their given time.

Goals are statements of intent, such as learning to walk again or to drive a car. You need to establish activities (i.e., courses of action) in order to meet your goals. These might include physical therapy on a daily basis, exercising, or taking proper medication. Establish priorities for your goals. Reexamine your goals to ensure that you are making progress. Constantly ask yourself, "Am I making the best use of my time right now?" This will help monitor your progress.

Reward yourself for your progress. Everyone enjoys positive reinforcement (i.e., "strokes"). If others don't reinforce you, reinforce yourself. A child who had undergone surgery slowly progressed each day and during each step of the way was rewarded with a gold star. Although this reinforcement was quite simple, it was very powerful in reinforcing the child's determination.

## When Things Go Bad—It's Still Win/Win

Not all conditions result in having a good outcome. Sometimes people are left with chronic long-term pain and suffering, become incapacitated, or develop physical handicaps. Other times, healing takes place gradually rather than instantaneously. People respond differently. Some are able to compensate for their condition and make the best of it, while others let their illness handicap their entire life. Still, we must resign ourselves to the fact that there are no magic formulas for dealing with a bad result or with a terminal illness.

One of the most dreaded diseases of our time is AIDS— a cruel and merciless affliction. With this illness, as with other terminal illnesses, pray for compassion and mercy. God does not inflict evil. God is good. Recognize that God does not send disease to punish us. During a time of intense suffering, humiliation, loss of self-esteem, depression, loneliness, rejection, and suicidal thoughts are common as death nears. Victims feel guilt and shame as they become a medical and financial burden on their family and friends. Yet, God is merciful and through his eyes sees only the love relationship between him and his people. The separation between life here on earth and heaven is not seen in the same perspective by mortal humans. Our challenge is to provide comfort, care, and compassion to those with a terminal illness. The suffering patient is at the mercy of God and needs the compassion of humanity.

If you must contend with a terminal illness, approach the condition as a war between you and the disease. Pray to God for his healing and merciful blessing and remember that God will never let you down. Think of this war as always having a winning outcome. You always win in the end. It's a win/win situation. If you eradicate the disease through medical treatment or God's healing miracle, you win against the disease. But if you should die, this disease will be destroyed along with your physical body and you will be victorious as your spiritual soul lives on in heaven. You will always be ultimately victorious! "Where, O death, is your victory? Where, O death, is your sting?" (1 Cor. 15:55).

## Going on with Life

Never forget your crisis! Gain wisdom and grow from it. You may need to reconstruct your priorities in life. If you are left with a handicap, recognize that there are other positive things in life and that the disability is only one part of the whole. Don't let a handicap overpower you. Remember, no one can escape the ups and downs of life. Recognize that everyone, no matter who, will experience both positive and negative aspects to varying degrees. Eleanor Roosevelt said, "You gain strength, courage, and confidence by every experience in which you really stop to look fear in the face. You are able to say to yourself, 'I lived through this horror. I can take the next thing that comes along'. . . . You must do the thing you think you cannot do."

We have talked with many parents around the country who have also been faced with a brain tumor in their child, and all were determined to fight for their child's health. Many saw themselves in a personal battle against the tumor. Even when the condition was deemed terminal, they continued to explore as many avenues as possible so that they would be able to look back and know that they had done everything possible to help save their child's life.

Remember the power of high expectations and prayer: You often get what you expect. God does answer prayer. If you don't expect much, you won't get much. Therefore, if you expect the best, then your chances of obtaining the right doctor will be greater. Don't give up. Do everything that you possibly can in your search for the best doctor and the best medical treatment plan and you will never suffer guilt. Take charge of your medical care, be a wise health consumer, and exercise your options.

# *Appendix A*

## ORGANIZATIONS AND FOUNDATIONS

### AIDS

American Foundation for AIDS
Research
5900 Wilshire Blvd.
Los Angeles, CA 90036
213-857-5900

Gay Men's Health Crisis
129 W. 20th St.
New York, NY 10011
212-807-6664

Pediatric AIDS Coalition
1331 Pennsylvania Ave., NW
Suite 721-N
Washington, DC
202-662-7460

People with AIDS Coalition
31 W. 26th St.
New York, NY 10010
212-532-0290

Ryan White National Fund
(AIDS)
Nissan Motor Corp.
PO Box 191
Gardena, CA 90248-0191
213-768-8493

San Francisco AIDS Foundation
PO Box 6182

San Francisco, CA 94101
415-864-5855

### Alcoholism and Drug Dependency

Do It Now Foundation
Institute for Chemical Survival
PO Box 5115
Phoenix, AZ 85010
602-491-0393

Hazelden Foundation
PO Box 11
Center City, MN 55012
800-238-9000

Narcotics Anonymous
16155 Wyandotte St.
Van Nuys, CA 91406
818-780-3951

National Council on Alcoholism
12 W. 21st St., 7th floor
New York, NY 10010
212-206-6770

### Allergy and Asthma *(also see Immunology)*

Allergy Foundation of America
1835 K St., NW
Suite P-900

Washington, DC 20006
202-293-2950

American Academy of Allergy
and Immunology
611 E. Wells St.
Milwaukee, WI 53202
414-272-6074

American Allergy Association
PO Box 7277
Merlo, CA 94026
415-322-1663

American College of Allergy
and Immunology
800 E. N.W. Highway
Suite 1080
Palatine, IL 60067
708-359-2800

Asthma and Allergy Foundation
1717 Massachusetts NE
Suite 305
Washington, DC 20036
202-265-0265

Asthmatic Children's Foundation
of NY
PO Box 568
Ossing, NY 10562
914-762-2110

## Alzheimer's Disease

Alzheimer's Disease
International
70 E. Lake St., Suite 600
Chicago, IL 60601
312-853-3060

## Amputation

National Amputation Foundation
12–45 150th St.

Whitestone, NY 11357
718-767-0596

## Anemia *(see Blood)*

## Anorexia *(see Eating Disorders)*

## Anesthesiology and Respiratory

American Society of
Anesthesiologists
575 Busse Highway
Park Ridge, IL 60068
312-825-5586

## Arteriosclerosis *(see Heart)*

## Arthritis *(also see Endocrinology, Orthopedics or Hand)*

American Rheumatic Association
17 Executive Park Dr., NE
Atlanta, GA 30329
404-633-3777

Arthritis Foundation
1314 Spring St., NW
Atlanta, GA 30309
404-872-7100

## Asthma *(see Allergy)*

## Attention Deficit Syndrome

Attention Deficit Syndrome
499 NW 70th Ave, Suite 308
Plantation, FL 33317
305-587-3700

## Autism

Autism Services Center
Douglass Ed. Building
10th Ave. & Bruce St.

Huntington, WV 25701
304-525-8014

Autism Society of America
8601 Georgia, Suite 503
Silver Springs, MD 20910
301-565-0433

**Back** *(see Neurology, Pain, Orthopedics, or Spine)*

**Birth Defects**

Association of Children's Birth Defects
Orlando Executive Park
5400 Diplomat Circle
Suite 270
Orlando, FL 32810
407-629-1466

Cornelia DeLange Syndrome Foundation
60 Dyer Ave.
Collingsville, CT 06022
203-693-0159

March of Dimes Birth Defects Foundation
1275 Mamar-Oneck Ave.
White Plains, NY 10605
914-428-7100

**Blindness** *(see Eyes)*

**Blood** *(Hematology)*

American Association of Blood Banks
1117 N. 19th St., Suite 600
Arlington, VA 22209
703-528-8200

Blood Club
National Rare Blood Center
Associated Health Foundation

164 5th Avenue
New York, NY 10010
212-243-8037

Cooley's Anemia Foundation
105 E. 22nd St., Suite 911
New York, NY 10010
212-598-0911

Fanconi's Anemia
66 Club Rd., Suite 390
Eugene, OR 97401
503-687-4658

**Blood Pressure** *(see Heart)*

**Bone Marrow Transplants**

University of Washington
Affiliated Hospitals
1959 NE Pacific St.
Seattle, WA 98195
206-543-3300
206-543-8856

**Bones** *(also see Orthopedics)*

American Brittle Bones Society
1256 Merrill Dr.
West Chester, PA 19382
215-692-6248

National Osteoporosis Foundation (NOF)
2100 M St., NW, Suite 602
Washington, DC 20037
202-223-2226

**Brain Tumors** *(also see Children and Neurosurgery)*

Accoustic Neuroma Association
PO Box 398
Carlisle, PA 17013
717-249-4783

Association for Brain Tumor
Research
6232 N. Pulaski Rd.
Chicago, IL 60646
312-286-5571
312-984-1000

American Brain Tumor
Association
3725 N. Talman Ave.
Chicago, IL 60618
312-286-5571
800-886-2282

Brain Tumor Foundation
for Children
751 DeKalb
Decatur, GA 30033
404-292-0395

Brain Tumor Society
258 Harvard St., Suite 308
Brookline, MA 02146
617-243-4229

National Brain Tumor
Foundation
323 Geary St., Suite 510
San Francisco, CA 94102
415-296-0404

**Breast** *(see Plastic Surgery
and Cancer)*

**Burns**

National Burn Victim
Foundation
308 Man St.
Orange, NJ 07050
201-731-3112

**Cancer**

American Cancer Society
777 Third

New York, NY 10017
212-371-2900

American Society of Clinical
Oncology
435 N. Michigan, Suite 1717
Chicago, IL 60611
312-644-0828

Candle Fighters
123 C St., SW
Washington, DC 20003
202-483-9100

Candlelighters Childhood
Cancer Foundation
1312 18th St., NW, Suite 200
Washington, DC 20036-1808
800-366-CCCF
202-659-5136

National Alliance of Breast
Cancer Organizations (NABCO)
1180 Avenue of the Americas
2nd Floor
New York, NY 10036
212-719-0154

National Cancer Institute
9000 Rockville Pike, Bldg. 31
Bethesda, MD 20205
301-496-5583
800-4-CANCER

Skin Cancer Foundation
245 5th Ave., Suite 2402
New York, NY 10016
212-725-5176

**Cerebral Palsy**

United Cerebral Palsy
Association
7 Penn Plaza, Suite 804

New York, NY 10001
212-268-6655

**Chest** *(see Thoracic)*

**Children** *(Pediatrics)*

American Academy of Pediatrics
PO Box 927
Elk Grove Village, IL 60009-
0937
708-228-5005

Association for Care of
Children's Health
7910 Woodmont Ave.,
Suite 300
Bethesda, MD 20814
301-654-6549

American Society for Pediatric
Neurosurgery
c/o M. L. Walker
100 N. Medical Ctr.
Salt Lake City, UT 84113
801-588-3400

**Chiropractic** *(see Joint Manipulation)*

**Cleft Palate** *(see Plastic Surgery)*

**Colon** *(see Cancer, Diseases, or Proctology)*

**Crippled Children**

Crippled Children
Shriners' Hospital
2900 Rock Point Dr.
Tampa, FL 33607
813-281-0300
800-237-5055

**Dental**

American Dental Association
211 E. Chicago Ave.
Chicago, IL 60611
312-440-2500

American Society of Dentistry
for Children
211 E. Chicago Ave.
Chicago, IL 60611
312-440-2500

**Dermatology** *(see Skin)*

**Diabetes**

American Diabetes Association
1660 Duke St.
Alexandria, VA 22314
703-549-1500

National Diabetes Information
Clearinghouse
Box NDIC
Bethesda, MD 20892
301-568-2162

**Digestive Disorders** *(See Internal Medicine)*

**Disabilities**

Information Center for
Individuals with Disabilities
20 Park Plaza, Room 330
Boston, MA 02116
617-727-5540

National Information Center for
Handicapped Children & Youth
(NICHY)
PO Box 1492
Washington, DC 20013
800-999-5599

**Diseases** *(Miscellaneous Diseases)*

American Behcet's Association
421 21st Ave., NW
Rochester, MN 55902
507-281-3059

Center for Disease Control
Bureau of Health Education
1600 Clifton Rd., NE
Atlanta, GA 30333
04-329-3534

Charcot-Marie-Tooth Association
c/o C. Mills
600 Upland Ave.
Upland, PA 19105
215-499-7486

Colitis and Ileitis Foundation
444 Park Ave.
New York, NY 10016
212-685-3440

Cystic Fibrosis Foundation
6931 Arlington Rd., No. 200
Bethesda, MD 20814
301-951-4422

Fibrositis Association
Riverside Hospital
N. Medical Bldg., Suite 8
3545 Olentangy River Rd.
Columbus, OH 43214
614-262-8020

Friedeich's Adaxia Group
PO Box 11116
Oakland, CA 94611
415-655-0833

Huntington's Disease Society of America
140 W. 22nd St., 6th floor

New York, NY 10040
212-242-1968

Iron Overload Association
224 Datura St., Suite 912
West Palm Beach, FL 33401
305-659-5616

Laurence-Moon Bardot Biedl Syndrome
2622 Cockrell Ave.
Ft. Worth, TX 76109
817-924-8594

Lowe's Syndrome Association
222 Lincoln St.
West Lafayette, IN 47906
317-743-3634

Lyme Disease
PO Box 462
Tolland, CT 06084
203-871-2900

Marfan Foundation
382 Main St.
Port Washington, NY 11050
516-883-8712

Muscular Dystrophy Association
810 7th Ave.
New York, NY 10017
212-586-0808

Myasthena Gravis Foundation
53 W. Jackson Blvd, Suite 1352
Chicago, IL 60604
312-427-6252

National Association for Sickle Cell Disease
3345 Wilshire Blvd., Suite 1106
Los Angeles, CA 90010
213-736-5455

National Gaucher Foundation
(metabolic disorder)
1424 K St. NW, 4th floor
Washington, DC 20005
202-393-2777

National Organization
for Rare Disorders
PO Box 8923
New Fairfield, CT 06812
203-746-6518

Paget's Disease
PO Box 2772
Brooklyn, NY 11202
718-596-1043

Reyes Syndrome Association
426 N. Lewis
PO Box 829
Bryan, OH 43506
419-636-2679

Russell-Silver Syndrome
22 Hoyt St.
Madison, NJ 07940
201-377-4531

Spina Bifida Association
of America
1700 Rockville Pike, Suite 250
Rockville, MD 20852
301-770-SBAA
800-621-3141

Tay-Sachs Disease National
Association
385 Elliot St.
Newton, MA 02164
617-964-5508

Tourette Syndrome Association
42-40 Bell Blvd.
Bayside, NY 11361
718-224-2999

**Doctors** *(see Physicians)*

**Down's Syndrome**

National Association for
Down's Syndrome (NADS)
PO Box 4542
Oak Brook, IL 60522-4542
708-325-9112

National Down's Syndrome
Society (NDSS)
66 Broadway
New York, NY 10012
212-460-9330

**Drug Dependence** *(see*
*Alcoholism & Drug*
*Dependency)*

**Dyslexia**

Dyslexia Society
724 York Rd.
Baltimore, MD 21204
301-296-0232

**Ears** *(see Head, Hearing*
*Impaired, or*
*Otorhinolaryngology)*

**Eating Disorders**

Anorexia Nervosa & Related
Eating Disorders (ANRED)
PO Box 5102
Eugene, OR 97405
503-344-1144

National Anorexic Aid Society
5796 Karl Rd.
Columbus, OH 43229
614-436-1112

**Elbow** *(also see Orthopedics)*

American Shoulder & Elbow Surgeons (ASES)
222 S. Prospect Ave., Suite 127
Park Ridge, IL 60068
708-823-7186

**Endocrinology** *(also see Arthritis, Diabetes, Diseases, Internal Medicine, Lupus, or Thyroid)*

Endocrine Society
9650 Rockville Pike
Bethesda, MD 20814
301-571-1802

**Epilepsy**

Epilepsy Foundation of America
4531 Garden City Drive
Landover, MD 20785
301-459-3700

**Eyes**

American Academy of Ophthalmology
655 Beach St., Suite 300
San Francisco, CA 94109
415-561-8500

American Foundation
for the Blind, Inc.
15 W. 16th St.
New York, NY 10011
212-620-2000

Better Vision Institute
1800 N. Kent St., Suite 1210
Rosslyn, VA 22209
703-243-1508

Christian Record Braille Foundation

4444 S. 52nd St.
Lincoln, NE 68506
402-488-0981

National Eye Institute
National Institutes of Health
Building 10
Bethesda, MD 20205
301-496-3123

**Face** *(see Otorhinolaryngology, Neurology, Plastic Surgery or TMJ)*

**Fatigue**

Chronic Fatigue Syndrome Association
PO Box 230108
Portland, OR 97223
503-684-5261

**Feet (Podiatry)** *(also see Orthopedics)*

American Board of Podiatric Surgery
1601 Dolores St.
San Francisco, CA 94110
415-826-3200

American Orthopedic Foot and Ankle Society
222 S. Prospect Ave.
Park Ridge, IL 60068
708-698-1626

**Gall Bladder** *(see Diseases, Internal Medicine, or Liver)*

**Gastroenterology** *(stomach, intestine)*

American Gastroenterological Association

6900 Grove Rd.
Thorofare, NJ 08086
609-848-1000

## Genetic Disorders

National Foundation for
Genetic Disorders
219 E. Main, Box 114
Mascoutah, IL 62258
618-566-2020

## Geriatrics *(Senior Citizens, Aging)*

American Geriatrics Society
770 Lexington Ave., Suite 400
New York, NY 10021
212-308-1414

American Association of Homes
for Aging
1129 20th St., NW, Suite 400
Washington, DC 20036
202-296-5960

National Institute on Aging
9000 Rockville Pike
Building 31, Room 5C35
Bethesda, MD 20892
301-496-1752

## Glands *(see Diseases, Endocrinology, or Internal Medicine)*

## Goiter *(see Arthritis, Endocrinology, or Internal Medicine)*

## Gynecology *(see Obstetrics/Gynecology or Infertility)*

## Hand *(also see Neurosurgery or Orthopedics)*

Hand Surgery Association
2934 Fish Hatchery Rd.,

Suite 210
Madison, WI 53713
608-273-8940

International Federation of
Societies for Surgery of
the Hand
1900 Wealthy St. SE
Grand Rapids, MI 49506
616-774-0191

## Handicapped *(see Disabilities)*

## Head *(Injuries, Headaches, TMJ, or Trauma)*

Brain Research Foundation
208 S. LaSalle St., Suite 1426
Chicago, IL 60604
312-782-4311

National Head Injury
Foundation, Inc.
333 Turnpike Rd.
Southboro, MA 01772
508-485-9950
800-444-6443

National Headache Foundation
5252 N. Western Ave.
Chicago, IL 60625
312-878-7715

## Hearing Impaired

National Association
of the Deaf
814 Thayer St.
Silver Springs, MD 20910
301-587-1788

National Hearing Aid Society
20361 Middlebelt
Livonia, MI 48152
313-478-2610

## Heart (Arteriosclerosis, Cardiology, Hypertension, Vascular)

American College of Cardiology
9111 Old Georgetown Rd.
Bethesda, MD 20814
301-897-5400

American Heart Association
7320 Greenville Avenue
Dallas, TX 75231
214-373-6300

Heart Disease Research
Foundation
50 Court St.
Brooklyn, NY 11201
718-649-6210

High Blood Pressure
Information Center
120/80 National Institute
of Health
Bethesda, MD 20892
301-496-1809

## Herpes (see Sexually Transmitted Diseases)

## Hip (see Orthopedics)

## Hormones (see Diseases, Internal Medicine, or Obstetrics)

## Hospice

National Hospice Organization
1901 N. Fort Myer St.,
Suite 307
Arlington, VA 22209
703-243-5900
800-658-8898

## Hospitals

American Hospital Association
840 N. Lakeshore Dr.
Chicago, IL 60611
312-280-6000

National Association for Patient
Representation & Consumer
Affairs
PO Box 96003
Chicago, IL 60693
312-280-6426

## Hypertension (see Heart)

## Hydrocephalus (also see Brain Tumors)

Hydrocephalus Foundation
of Northern California
2040 Polk St., #342
San Francisco, CA 94109
415-776-4713

## Immunology (also see Allergy, Arthritis, Internal Medicine, or Gastroenterology)

Clinical Immunology Society
6900 Grove Rd.
Thorofare, NJ 08086
609-848-1000

## Infectious Diseases

National Foundation for
Infectious Diseases
4733 Bethesda Ave., Suite 750
Bethesda, MD 20814
301-656-0003

## Infertility (also see Obstetrics/Gynecology)

American Fertility Society (AFS)
2140 11th Ave. S., Suite 200

Birmingham, AL 35205-2800
205-933-8494

Fertility Research Foundation
(FRF)
1430 Second Ave., Suite 103
New York, NY 10021
212-744-5500

**Internal Medicine** *(also see Diseases, Endocrinology, Gastroenterology, Heart, Immunology, Kidney, Liver, Pulmonary, or Vascular)*

American Digestive Disease
Society
7720 Wisconsin Ave.
Bethesda, MD 20014
301-652-9293

**Joint Manipulation**

American Chiropractic
Association
1916 Wilson Blvd.
Arlington, VA 22201
703-276-8800

American Osteopathic
Association
142 E. Ontario St.
Chicago, IL 60601
312-280-5800

**Joints** *(see Orthopedics)*

**Kidney** *(nephrology)*

American Kidney Foundation
7315 Wisconsin
Bethesda, MD 20815
800-638-8299
301-986-1444

National Kidney Foundation
30E 33rd St., Suite 1100
New York, NY 10016
212-889-2210

**Knee** *(also see Orthopedics)*

International Society
of the Knee
70 W. Hubbard, Suite 202
Chicago, IL 60610
312-644-2623

**Larynx** *(also see Otorhinolaryngology)*

International Society of
Laryngectomies
219 E. 42nd St.
New York, NY 10017
212-867-3700

**Leukemia** *(also see Cancer)*

Leukemia Society of America
211 E. 43rd St.
New York, NY 10017
212-573-8484

Make Today Count, Inc.
PO Box 202
Burlington, IA 5260
319-754-7266
319-754-8977

National Leukemia Association
Roosevelt Field, Lower
Concourse
Garden City, NY 11530
516-741-1190

**Liver**

American Liver Foundation
1425 Compton Ave.

Cedar Grove, NJ 07005
201-256-2550

**Lung** *(Pulmonary, Respiratory)*

American Lung Association
1740 Broadway
New York, NY 10010
212-315-8700

**Lupus** *(also see Arthritis or Endocrinology)*

American Lupus Society
23751 Madison St.
Torrance, CA 90505
213-542-8891

Lupus Foundation of America
1717 Massachusetts Ave.
Washington, DC 20036
202-328-4550

Lupus Network
230 Ranch Dr.
Bridgeport, CT 06606
203-372-5792

**Mental Health**

American Association
of Mental Deficiency
1719 Kalorama Rd., NW
Washington, DC 20009
202-387-1968

American Psychiatric
Association, Inc.
1400 K St., NW
Washington, DC 20005
202-955-7600

American Psychological
Association
1200 17th St., NW

Washington, DC 20036
202-682-6000

Association for
Retarded Citizens
PO Box 6109
Arlington, TX 76005
817-640-0204

National Mental Health
Association (NMHA)
1021 Prince St.
Alexandria, VA 22314-2971
703-684-7722

National Alliance for
the Mentally Ill (NAMI)
2101 Wilson Blvd., Suite 302
Arlington, VA 22201
703-524-7600

**Multiple Sclerosis**

Multiple Sclerosis Society
205 E. 42nd St.
New York, NY 10017
212-986-3240

**Muscles** *(see Arthritis, Diseases, Neurology, Orthopedics, or Rehabilitation)*

**Neck** *(see Neurology, Orthopedics, Pain, or TMJ)*

**Nerves** *(see Diseases, Neurology, Orthopedics, or Pain)*

**Neurology and Neurosurgery** *(also see Brain Tumors, Children, Orthopedics, or Spine)*

American Academy of
Neurology

2221 University Ave., Suite 335
Minneapolis, MN 55414
612-623-8115

American Association of
Neurological Surgeons
22 S. Washington, Suite 100
Park Ridge, IL 60068
708-692-9500

National Institute of
Neurological and
Communicative Disorders
and Stroke
National Institutes of Health
Building 31, Room 8A-06
Bethesda, MD 20205
301-496-5751

National Neurofibromatosis
Foundation
141 5th Ave., Suite 7-S
New York, NY 10070
212-460-8980

**Nose** *(see*
*Otorhinolaryngology or*
*Plastic Surgery)*

**Obstetrics/Gynecology**

American College of
Obstetricians and Gynecologists
409 12th St., SW
Washington, DC 20024
202-638-5577

American Society for
Psychoprophylaxis in Obstetrics
1840 Wilson Blvd., Suite 204
Arlington, VA 22201
703-524-7802

**Organs**

Human Neurospecimen Bank
VA Wadsworth Hospital Center
Los Angeles, CA 90073
213-824-4307
213-478-3711

International Society for
Artificial Organs (ISAO)
8937 Euclid Ave.
Cleveland, OH 44106
216-421-0757

The Brain Tissue Resource
Center
McLean Hospital
Belmont, MA 02178
617-855-2400

**Orthopedics** *(also see Bone)*

American Academy of
Orthopedic Surgeons
222 S. Prospect Avenue
Park Ridge, IL 60068
708-823-7186

**Ophthamology** *(see Eye)*

**Osteoporosis** *(see Bone,*
*Endocrinology or*
*Orthopedics)*

**Otology** *(see*
*Otorhinolaryngology)*

**Otorhinolaryngology** *(ENT:*
*Ears, Nose, Throat)*

American Academy of
Otolaryngic Allergy
8455 Colesville Rd., Suite 745
Silver Springs, MD 20910
301-588-1800

American Laryngological
Rhinological & Otological
Society
c/o Lillibet Coe
PO Box 155
East Greenville, PA 18041
215-679-7180

## Pain

International Association for
Study of Pain (IASP)
909 NE 43rd, Suite 306
Seattle, WA 98105

Traditional Acupuncture
Institute
American City Building,
Suite 100
Columbia, MD 21044
301-596-6006

**Pancreas** *(see Diseases or
Internal Medicine)*

**Parkinson's Disease**

American Parkinson's Disease
60 Bay St., Suite 401
Staten Island, NY 10301
212-981-8001

American Parkinson's Disease
Association
147 E. 50th St.
New York, NY 10022
212-732-9550

National Parkinson Foundation
1501 NW 9th
Miami, FL 33136
305-547-6666

**Phobias**

Phobia Society
133 Rollins Ave., Suite 4-B
Rockville, MD 20852
301-231-5484

**Pituitary** *(also see Brain
Tumors, Endocrinology, or
Neurosurgery)*

Human Growth Foundation
7777 Leesburg Pike
Falls Church, VA 22043
703-883-1773

**Physicians**

American Medical Association
535 N. Dearborn St.
Chicago, IL 60601
312-464-5000

**Plastic & Reconstructive
Surgery**

American Academy of Facial
and Reconstructive Surgery
1110 Vermont Ave., NW,
Suite 220
Washington, DC 20005
202-842-4500

American Society of Plastic and
Reconstructive Surgery
444 E. Algonquin Rd.
Arlington Heights, IL 60005
708-228-9900

Cleft Palate-Craniofacial
Association
1218 Grandview Ave.
Pittsburgh, PA 15211
412-481-1376

**Podiatry** *(see Feet)*

**Proctology**

American Society of Colon and
Rectal Surgeons
800 E. Northwest Hwy,
Suite 1080
Palatine, IL 60067
708-359-9184

**Psychology** *(see Mental Health)*

**Pulmonary** *(see Internal Medicine, or Lung)*

**Rectum** *(see Proctology)*

**Reflex Sympathetic Dystrophy** *(also see Neurology or Orthopedics)*

Reflex Sympathetic Dystrophy
Association
PO Box 821
Haddonfield, NJ 08033
215-955-5444

**Rehabilitation**

American Academy of Physical
Medicine & Rehabilitation
122 S. Michigan Ave.,
Suite 1300
Chicago, IL 60603
312-922-9366

National Easter Seal Society
2023 W. Ogdon Ave.
Chicago, IL 60612
312-243-8400

**Rheumatism** *(see Arthritis, Endocrinology, Hand, or Orthopedics)*

**Rhinology** *(see Otorhinolaryngology)*

**Scleroderma** *(see Arthritis, Skin, or Vascular)*

**Scoliosis** *(also see Orthopedics)*

Scoliosis Research Society
222 S. Prospect Ave., Suite 127
Park Ridge, IL 60068
708-698-1628

**Senior Citizens** *(see Geriatrics)*

**Sexual Disorders** *(also see Obstetrics)*

Impotence Institute of America
119 S. Ruth St.
Maryville, TN 37801
615-983-6064

Sex Therapy Society (SSTAR)
c/o Dr. R. Taylor Segraves
19910 S. Woodland
Shaker Heights, OH 44122
216-459-3634

**Sexually Transmitted Diseases**

American Social Health
Association
PO Box 13827
Research Triangle Park, NC
27709
919-361-8400

American Venereal Disease
Association

PO Box 1753
Baltimore, MD 21203-1753
301-955-3150

Herpes Resource Center (HRC)
PO Box 13827
Research Triangle Park, NC
27709
919-361-2120

## Shoulder (also see Elbow and Orthopedics)

## Skin

American College of
Dermatology
1567 Maple Ave.
PO Box 3116
Evanston, IL 60201
708-869-3954

Dermatology Foundation (DF)
1560 Sherman Ave.
Evanston, IL 60201
708-328-2256

Ehlers Danlos Foundation
(Fragile Skin)
PO Box 1212
Southgate, MI 48195
313-282-0180

Scleroderma Foundation
PO Box 350
Watsonville, CA 95077
408-728-2202

## Sleep Disorders (Narcolepsy)

American Narcolepsy
Association
PO Box 1187

San Carlos, CA 94070
415-591-7979

Association of Sleep Disorders
PO Box 2604
Del Mar, CA 92014
619-755-7556

## Speech

American Speech Language
Hearing Association
10801 Rockville Pike
Rockville, MD 20852
301-897-5700

## Spine (also see Joint Manipulation, Neurosurgery, Orthopedics, or Pain)

National Spinal Cord Injury
Association
600 W. Cummings Park,
Suite 2000
Woburn, MA 01801
617-935-2722

North American Spine Society
222 S. Prospect
Park Ridge, IL 60068
708-698-1628

## Stomach (see Digestive, Gastroenterology, or Internal Medicine)

## Stroke (also see Neurology)

National Stroke Association
300 E. Hampton Ave.,
Suite 240
Englewood, CO 80110
303-762-9922

## Sudden Infant Death Syndrome (SIDS)

National Sudden Infant Death Syndrome Foundation (NSIDSF)
10500 Little Patuxent Parkway, No. 420
Columbia, MD 21044
301-964-8000

**Synovitis** *(see Arthritis or Orthopedics)*

**Teeth** *(see Dental)*

**Thoracic** *(also see Heart)*

American Association of Thoracic Surgery
13 Elm St., PO Box 1565
Manchester, MA 01944
508-526-8330

American College of Chest Physicians
922 Busse Highway
Park Ridge, IL 60068
708-498-1400

**Thyroid** *(also see Endocrinology)*

Thyroid Association
Walter Reed Army
Medical Center
Endocrine-Metabolic Service
Washington, DC 20307
202-882-7717

## TMJ

American Academy of Head, Facial & Neck Pain & TMJ Orthopedics
Atlanta Bldg., Suite 1310
360 S. Broad St.
Philadelphia, PA 19102
215-545-2100

**Tumors** *(see Cancer and Specialty Area)*

## Urology

American Urological Association
1120 N. Charles St.
Baltimore, MD 21201
301-727-1100

**Vascular** *(also see Heart)*

American College of Angiology
1044 Northern Blvd., Suite 103
Roslyn, NY 11576
516-484-6880

**Venereal Disease** *(see Sexually Transmitted Diseases)*

# *Appendix B*

## HOTLINE SERVICES

| | |
|---|---|
| AIDS Hotline | 1-800-343-AIDS |
| | 1-800-447-AIDS |
| | 1-800-AID-AIDS |
| | 1-800-544-0586 |
| | 1-212-807-6655 |
| Alzheimer Disease | 1-800-272-3900 |
| American Hair Loss Hotline | 1-800-274-8717 |
| Asthma | 1-800-222-LUNG |
| American Brain Tumor Association | 1-800-886-2282 |
| American Cancer Society Helpline | 1-800-ACS-2345 |
| Autism National Hotline | 1-304-525-8026 |
| Blindness | 1-900-424-8567 |
| Brain Damage | 1-800-445-8106 |
| Brain Tumor Information Service | 1-312-799-8228 |
| Brain Tumors | 1-800-886-2282 |
| Brain Tumors/Cancer | 1-800-366-CCCF |
| Breast Cancer Hotline | 1-312-799-8228 |
| Cancer Consulting Group, Nationwide Networking | 1-312-866-7711 |
| Cancer Hotline | 1-816-932-8463 |
| Cancer Information Service | 1-800-4-CANCER |
|    Alabama | 1-800-292-6201 |
|    Alaska | 1-800-638-6070 |
|    California | 1-800-252-9066 |
|    Connecticut | 1-800-922-0824 |
|    Delaware | 1-800-523-3586 |
|    District of Columbia (includes suburbs in Maryland & Virginia) | 202-623-5700 |
|    Florida | 1-800-432-5953 |
|    Georgia | 1-800-327-7332 |

212

| | |
|---|---|
| Hawaii, Oahu (neighboring islands, ask operator for Enterprise 6702) | 808-524-1234 |
| Illinois | 1-800-972-0586 |
| Kentucky | 1-800-432-9321 |
| Maine | 1-800-225-7034 |
| Maryland | 1-800-492-1444 |
| Massachusetts | 1-800-952-7420 |
| Michigan | 1-800-482-4959 |
| Minnesota | 1-800-582-5262 |
| New Hampshire | 1-800-225-7034 |
| New Jersey | |
| (Northern) | 1-800-223-1000 |
| (Southern) | 1-800-523-3586 |
| New York State | 1-800-462-7255 |
| New York City | 1-212-794-7982 |
| North Carolina | 1-800-672-0943 |
| North Dakota | 1-800-328-5188 |
| Ohio | 1-800-282-6422 |
| Pennsylvania | 1-800-822-3963 |
| South Dakota | 1-800-328-5188 |
| Texas | 1-800-392-2040 |
| Vermont | 1-800-225-7034 |
| Washington | 1-800-552-7212 |
| Wisconsin | 1-800-362-8038 |
| All other areas | 1-800-638-6694 |
| Cancer PDQ System | 1-800-422-6237 |
| Children's Disease | 1-800-237-5055 |
| Crippled Children (Shriners) | 1-800-237-5055 |
| Cystic Fibrosis | 1-800-FIGHT-CF |
| Data Bank (Health Professionals only) | 1-800-767-6732 |
| Deaf and Hearing-Impaired | 1-800-243-7889 |
| Diabetes Association | 1-900-232-3472 |
| Digestive Disorders | 1-800-652-9293 |
| Down's Syndrome Society | 1-800-221-4602 |
| Dyslexia | 1-800-ABC-D123 |
| Drug and Alcohol Dependency | 1-800-COCAINE |
| | 1-800-328-9000 |
| | 1-800-662-HELP |
| Emily Snider Cancer Helpline | 1-815-758-1144 |
| Epilepsy Foundation | 1-800-EFA-1000 |

| | |
|---|---|
| Eye Donation Hotline | 1-800-638-1818 |
| Head Injury | 1-800-444-6443 |
| Hearing Problems | 1-800-638-TALK |
| | 1-800-424-8576 |
| Hearing Aid Hotline | 1-800-521-5247 |
| Heart Disorders | 1-800-241-6993 |
| Hospice Help Line | 1-800-658-8898 |
| Kidney Disease | 1-800-638-8299 |
| Lung Disorders | 1-800-222-LUNG |
| Lupus Foundation of America | 1-800-558-0121 |
| National Autism Hotline | 304-525-8026 |
| National Organization of Rare Diseases | 1-800-999-NORD |
| Organ Donations | 1-800-872-2971 |
| Parkinson's Disease | 1-800-344-7872 |
| | 1-800-250-2975 |
| Phobias | 1-800-332-7359 |
| Surgical Opinion Hotline | 1-800-638-6833 |
| (in Maryland) | 1-800-492-6603 |
| VD National Hotline | 1-800-227-8922 |

# *Appendix C*

## CONSULTING GROUPS AND FEDERAL HEALTH SERVICES

AIDS Clinical Trials Group
c/o Maureen Myers
National Institute of Health
6003 Executive Blvd., Room 200P
Rockville, MD 20852
301-496-8210

AIDS National Clearinghouse
(NAIC)
PO Box 6003
Rockville, MD
    Computerized Data Bank
    800-243-7012
    800-458-5231
    301-217-0023

Alcohol and Drug Abuse
National Institute
Parklawn Building
5600 Fishers Lane
Rockville, MD 20857

Cancer Consulting Group, Inc.
One American Plaza
Evanston, IL 60201
312-866-7711

Center for Medical Consumers
237 Thompson St.

New York, New York 10012
212-674-7105

Center for Disease Control
Building 1 R B63
1600 Clifton Rd. N.E.
Atlanta, GA 30333

Experimental Therapies
The Clinical Center
Building 10, Room 2c-146
National Institute of Health
Bethesda, MD 20892

Health Research Group
2000 P St., NW
Washington, DC 20036
202-872-0320

National Cancer Institute
PDQ Computer System
Building 82, Room 121A
Bethesda, MD 20892
800-422-6232
301-480-8105

National Organization for
Rare Disorders
Data Bank
PO Box 8923
New Fairfield, CT 06812
203-746-6518

215

Office of Consumer and
Professional Affairs
5600 Fishers Lane
Rockville, MD 20857

Office of Scientific and Health
Reports
NIH-NINOS
9000 Rockville Pike
Building 31, Room 8A-16
Bethesda, MD 20892
301-296-5751

Peoples Medical Society
462 Walnut St.
Allentown, PA 18102

Planetree Health Resource
Center

2040 Webster St.
San Francisco, CA 94115
415-923-3680

The Health Resource
209 Katherine Dr.
Conway, AR 72032
501-329-5272

U.S. Department of Health &
Human Services
Public Health Service &
Inquiries
National Institute of Health
9000 Rockville Pike
Bethesda, MD 20892
301-496-5583

# Appendix D
## *AMERICA'S BEST HOSPITALS
## MEDICAL SURVEY

†The Best of the Best

JOHNS HOPKINS HOSPITAL
Baltimore, MD
13 Specialties

MAYO CLINIC
Rochester, MN
12 Specialties

MASSACHUSETTS GENERAL
Boston, MA
11 Specialties

UCLA MEDICAL CENTER
Los Angeles, CA
9 Specialties

CLEVELAND CLINIC
Cleveland, OH
5 Specialties

DUKE UNIVERSITY
MEDICAL CENTER
Durham, NC
4 Specialties

MEMORIAL SLOAN-
KETTERING CANCER
CENTER
New York, NY
4 Specialties

UNIVERSITY OF TEXAS
(M.D. Anderson Cancer Center)
Houston, TX
4 specialties

STANFORD UNIVERSITY
HOSPITAL
Stanford, CA
3 Specialties

UNIVERSITY OF
CALIFORNIA
SAN FRANCISCO
MEDICAL CENTER
San Francisco, CA
3 Specialties

### AIDS

UNIVERSITY OF
CALIFORNIA
SAN FRANCISCO GENERAL
HOSPITAL / 61%

*America's Best Hospitals. Copyright June 15, 1992, *U. S. News & World Report.*

†These hospitals appear on at least three of the 16 specialty lists in the *U. S. News* Survey.

MASSACHUSETTS GENERAL HOSPITAL
Boston / 27%

JOHNS HOPKINS HOSPITAL
Baltimore / 22%

UCLA MEDICAL CENTER
Los Angeles /18%

UNIVERSITY OF CALIFORNIA
SAN FRANCISCO MEDICAL CENTER / 16%

MEMORIAL SLOAN-KETTERING CANCER CENTER
New York / 14%

CLINICAL CENTER
National Institutes of Health
Bethesda / 12%

## †The Best Hospitals for Specialty

### CANCER

UNIVERSITY OF TEXAS
(M.D. Anderson Cancer Center)
Houston / 62%

MEMORIAL SLOAN-KETTERING CANCER CENTER
New York / 57%

DAN-FARBER CANCER INSTITUTE
Boston / 36%

MAYO CLINIC
Rochester, MN / 23%

STANFORD UNIVERSITY HOSPITAL
Stanford / 22%

### CARDIOLOGY

MAYO CLINIC
Rochester, MN / 38%

CLEVELAND CLINIC
Ohio / 36%

TEXAS HEART INSTITUTE
(St. Luke's Episcopal Hospital)
Houston / 21%

STANFORD UNIVERSITY HOSPITAL
Stanford / 20%

MASSACHUSETTS GENERAL HOSPITAL
Boston / 19%

EMORY UNIVERSITY HOSPITAL
Atlanta / 16%

JOHNS HOPKINS HOSPITAL
Baltimore / 14%

### ENDOCRINOLOGY

MAYO CLINIC
Rochester, MN / 63%

MASSACHUSETTS GENERAL HOSPITAL
Boston / 62%

CLINICAL CENTER
NATIONAL INSTITUTES OF HEALTH
Bethesda / 32%

UNIVERSITY OF CALIFORNIA
SAN FRANCISCO MEDICAL CENTER / 26%

JOHNS HOPKINS HOSPITAL
Baltimore / 24%

BARNES HOSPITAL
St. Louis / 20%

## GASTROENTEROLOGY

MAYO CLINIC
Rochester, MN / 42%

MASSACHUSETTS GENERAL
HOSPITAL
Boston / 35% *ADL

CLEVELAND CLINIC
Ohio 31%

JOHNS HOPKINS HOSPITAL
Baltimore / 24%

UCLA MEDICAL CENTER
Los Angeles / 20%

MOUNT SINAI MEDICAL
CENTER
New York / 20%

## GERIATRICS

UCLA MEDICAL CENTER
Los Angeles / 22%

BETH ISRAEL HOSPITAL
Boston / 21%

DUKE UNIVERSITY
MEDICAL CENTER
Durham, NC / 18%

MOUNT SINAI MEDICAL
CENTER
New York / 16%

MASSACHUSETTS GENERAL
HOSPITAL
Boston / 14%

JOHNS HOPKINS HOSPITAL
Baltimore / 10%

## GYNECOLOGY

BRIGHAM AND WOMEN'S
HOSPITAL
Boston / 14%

JOHNS HOPKINS HOSPITAL
Baltimore / 14%

MAYO CLINIC
Rochester, MN / 13%

UNIVERSITY OF TEXAS
M. D. Anderson Cancer Center
Houston / 11%

DUKE UNIVERSITY
MEDICAL CENTER
Durham, N.C. / 9%

MASSACHUSETTS GENERAL
HOSPITAL
Boston / 8%

YALE-NEW HAVEN
HOSPITAL
New Haven, CT / 7%

MEMORIAL SLOAN-
KETTERING CANCER
CENTER
New York / 6%

## NEUROLOGY

MAYO CLINIC
Rochester, MN / 60%

MASSACHUSETTS GENERAL
HOSPITAL
Boston / 49%

JOHNS HOPKINS HOSPITAL
Baltimore / 39%

CLEVELAND CLINIC
Ohio / 36%

COLUMBIA-PRESBYTERIAN
MEDICAL CENTER
New York / 31%

UNIVERSITY OF
CALIFORNIA
SAN FRANCISCO MEDICAL
CENTER / 28%

UCLA MEDICAL CENTER
Los Angeles / 19%

## OPHTHALMOLOGY

JOHNS HOPKINS HOSPITAL
(WILMER EYE INSTITUTE)
Baltimore / 64%

BASCOM PALMER EYE
INSTITUTE
(UNIVERSITY OF MIAMI)
Miami / 55%

WILLS EYE HOSPITAL
Philadelphia / 42%

MASSACHUSETTS EYE AND
EAR INFIRMARY
Boston / 35%

UCLA MEDICAL CENTER
JULES STEIN EYE
INSTITUTE
Los Angeles / 28%

UNIVERSITY OF IOWA
HOSPITALS
Iowa City / 18%

## ORTHOPEDICS

HOSPITAL FOR SPECIAL
SURGERY
New York / 41%

MASSACHUSETTS GENERAL
HOSPITAL
Boston / 35%

MAYO CLINIC
Rochester, MN / 29%

DUKE UNIVERSITY
MEDICAL CENTER
Durham / 22%

JOHNS HOPKINS HOSPITAL
Baltimore / 19%

CLEVELAND CLINIC
Ohio / 16%

## OTOLARYNGOLOGY

UNIVERSITY OF IOWA
HOSPITALS AND CLINICS
Iowa City / 30%

MASSACHUSETTS EYE AND
EAR INFIRMARY
Boston / 26%

JOHNS HOPKINS HOSPITAL
Baltimore / 21%

UCLA MEDICAL CENTER
Los Angeles / 20%

MAYO CLINIC
Rochester, MN / 18% AD1
UNIVERSITY OF TEXAS (M.
D. Anderson Cancer Center
Houston / 18%

UNIVERSITY OF MICHIGAN
MEDICAL CENTER
Ann Arbor / 17%

## PEDIATRICS

CHILDREN'S HOSPITAL
Boston / 48%

CHILDREN'S HOSPITAL OF
PHILADELPHIA / 38%

JOHNS HOPKINS HOSPITAL
Baltimore / 29%

CHILDREN'S HOSPITAL
Los Angeles / 14%

RAINBOW BABIES AND
CHILDREN'S
HOSPITAL (UNIVERSITY
HOSPITALS
OF CLEVELAND) / 12%

## PSYCHIATRY

McLEAN HOSPITAL
Belmont, MA / 22%

MENNINGER CLINIC
Topeka / 18%

UCLA MEDICAL CENTER
Los Angeles / 15%

MASSACHUSETTS GENERAL
HOSPITAL
Boston / 14%

SHEPPARD AND ENOCH
PRATT HOSPITAL
Baltimore / 13%

INSTITUTE OF LIVING
Hartford, CT / 12%

MAYO CLINIC
Rochester, MN / 11%

COLUMBIA-PRESBYTERIAN
MEDICAL CENTER
New York / 10%

NEW YORK HOSPITAL-
CORNELL MEDICAL CENTER
New York / 10%

YALE-NEW HAVEN
HOSPITAL
New Haven, CT / 9%

## REHABILITATION

REHABILITATION
INSTITUTE
OF CHICAGO / 51%

UNIVERSITY OF
WASHINGTON MEDICAL
CENTER
Seattle / 46%

MAYO CLINIC
Rochester, MN / 31%

CRAIG HOSPITAL
Englewood, CO / 31%

INSTITUTE FOR
REHABILITATION AND
RESEARCH (TIRR)
Houston / 26%

RUSK INSTITUTE FOR
REHABILITATION
MEDICINE
(New york University Medical
Center)
New York / 26%

RANCHO LOS AMIGOS
MEDICAL CENTER
Downey, Calif. / 18%

## RHEUMATOLOGY

MAYO CLINIC
Rochester, MN / 46%

HOSPITAL FOR SPECIAL
SURGERY
New York / 27%

BRIGHAM AND WOMEN'S
HOSPITAL
Boston / 26%

UCLA MEDICAL CENTER
Los Angeles / 24%

JOHNS HOPKINS HOSPITAL
Baltimore / 16%

UNIVERSITY OF ALABAMA
HOSPITAL
Birmingham / 15%

MASSACHUSETTS GENERAL
HOSPTIAL
Boston 15%

## UROLOGY

MAYO CLINIC
Rochester, MN / 43%

JOHNS HOPKINS HOSPITAL
Baltimore / 38%

UCLA MEDICAL CENTER
Los Angeles 25%

CLEVELAND CLINIC
Ohio / 24%

MASSACHUSETTS GENERAL
HOSPITAL
Boston / 21%

DUKE UNIVERSITY
MEDICAL CENTER
Durham, NC 20%

UNIVERSITY OF TEXAS
(M. D. Anderson Cancer
Center)
Houston / 16%

MEMORIAL SLOAN-
KETTERING CANCER
CENTER
New York / 13%

STANFORD UNIVERSITY
HOSPITAL
California 10%

UNIVERSITY OF
WASHINGTON

MEDICAL CENTER / Seattle
9%

## A Guide to the Best

## NORTHEAST

BETH ISRAEL HOSPITAL
330 Brookline Avenue
Boston, MA 02215
(617) 735-2000
Best in: Intensive Care

BRIGHAM AND WOMEN'S
HOSPITAL
75 Francis Street
Boston, MA 02115
(617) 732-5500
Best in: Gynecology

CHILDREN'S HOSPITAL
300 Longwood Avenue
Boston, MA 02115
(617) 735-6000
Best in: Pediatrics

CHILDREN'S HOSPITAL OF
PHILADELPHIA
34th Street and Civic
Center Boulevard
Philadelphia, PA 19104
(215) 590-1000
Best in: Pediatrics

COLUMBIA-PRESBYTERIAN
MEDICAL CENTER
622 W. 168th Street
New York, NY 10032
(212) 305-2500
Best in: Neurology, psychiatry

DANA-FARBER CANCER
INSTITUTE
44 Binney Street
Boston, MA 02115

(617) 732-3000
Best in: Cancer

HOSPITAL FOR SPECIAL
SURGERY
535 East 70th Street
New York, NY 10021
(212) 606-1000
Best in: Orthopedics,
rheumatology

INSTITUTE OF LIVING
400 Washington Street
Hartford, CT 06106
(203) 241-8000
Best in: Psychiatry

MASSACHUSETTS EYE AND
EAR INFIRMARY
243 Charles Street
Boston, MA 02114
(617) 523-7900
Best in: Ophthalmology

MASSACHUSETTS GENERAL
HOSPITAL
55 Fruit Street
Boston, MA 02114
(617) 726-2000
Best in: AIDS, cardiology,
endocrinology, gastroenterology,
geriatrics, gynecology,
neurology, orthopedics,
psychiatry, rheumatology,
urology

McCLEAN HOSPITAL
115 Mill Street
Belmont, MA 02178
(617) 855-2000
Best in: Psychiatry

MEMORIAL SLOAN-
KETTERING CANCER

CENTER
1275 York Avenue
New York, NY 10021
(212) 639-2000
Best in: AIDS, cancer,
gynecology, urology

MOUNT SINAI MEDICAL
CENTER
1 Gustave L. Levy Place
New York, NY 10029
(212) 241-6500
Best in: Gastroenterology,
geriatrics

NEW YORK HOSPITAL-
CORNELL MEDICAL CENTER
525 East 68th Street
New York, NY 10021
(212) 746-5454
Best in: Psychiatry

RUSK INSTITUTE FOR
REHABILITATION
MEDICINE
400 East 34th Street
New York, NY 10016
(212) 263-7300
Best in: Rehabilitation

WILLS EYE HOSPITAL
900 Walnut Street
Philadelphia, PA 19107
(215) 928-3000
Best in: Ophthalmology

YALE-NEW HAVEN
HOSPITAL
20 York Street
New Haven, CT 06504
(203) 785-4242
Best in: Gynecology, psychiatry

## NORTH CENTRAL

**BARNES HOSPITAL**
1 Barnes Hospital Plaza
St. Louis, MO 63110
(314) 362-5000
Best in: Endocrinology

**CLEVELAND CLINIC**
One Clinic Center
9500 Euclid Avenue
Cleveland, OH 44195
(216) 444-2200
Best in: Cardiology,
gastroenterology, neurology,
orthopedics, urology

**MAYO CLINIC**
200 First Street N.W.
Rochester, MN 55905
(507) 284-2511
Best in: Cancer, cardiology,
endocrinology, gastroenterology,
gynecology, neurology,
orthopedics, otolaryngology,
psychiatry, rehabilitation,
rheumatology, urology

**MENNINGER CLINIC**
5800 W. Sixth Street
Topeka, KS 66606
(913) 273-7500
Best in: Pschiatry

**RAINBOW BABIES AND
CHILDREN'S HOSPITAL
(UNIVERSITY HOSPITALS
OF CLEVELAND)**
2074 Abington Road
Cleveland, OH 44106
(216) 844-1000
Best in: Pediatrics

**REHABILITATION
INSTITUTE OF CHICAGO**
345 East Superior Street
Chicago, IL 60611
(312) 908-6000
Best in: Rehabilitation

**UNIVERSITY OF IOWA
HOSPITALS AND CLINICS**
200 Hawkins Drive
Iowa City, IA 52242
(319) 356-1616
Best in: Ophthalmology,
otolaryngology

**UNIVERSITY OF MICHIGAN
HOSPITALS**
1500 East Medical Center Dr.
Ann Arbor, MI 48109
(313) 936-4000
Best in: Otolaryngology

## SOUTH

**BASCOM PALMER EYE
INSTITUTE
(UNIVERSITY OF MIAMI)**
900 N.W. 17th Street
Miami, FL 33136
(305) 326-6000
Best in: Ophthalmology

**CLINICAL CENTER,
NATIONAL
INSTITUTES OF HEALTH**
9000 Rockville Pike
Bethesda, MD 20892
(301) 496-4891
Best in: AIDS, endocrinology

**DUKE UNIVERSITY
MEDICAL CENTER**
Box 3708
Durham, NC 27704

(919) 684-8111
Best in: Geriatrics, gynecology,
orthopedics, urology

EMORY UNIVERSITY
HOSPITAL
1364 Clifton Road N.E.
Atlanta, GA 30322
(404) 727-7021
Best in: Cardiology

JOHNS HOPKINS HOSPITAL
(WILMER EYE INSTITUTE)
600 North Wolfe Street
Baltimore, MD 21205
(301) 955-5000
Best in: AIDS, cardiology,
endocrinology, gastroenterology,
geriatrics, gynecology,
neurology, ophthalmology,
orthopedics, otolaryngology,
pediatrics, rheumatology,
urology

SHEPPARD AND ENOCH
PRATT HOSPITAL
6501 N. Charles Street
Baltimore, MD 21204
(410) 938-3000
Best in: Psychiatry

TEXAS HEART INSTITUTE
(ST. LUKE'S EPISCOPAL
HOSPITAL)
6720 Bertner Avenue
Houston, TX 77030
(713) 791-2011
Best in: Cardiology

INSTITUTE FOR
REHABILITATION AND
RESEARCH (TIRR)
1333 Moursund Avenue

Houston, TX 77030
(713) 779-5000
Best in: Rehabilation

UNIVERSITY OF ALABAMA
HOSPITAL
619 S. 19th Street
Birmingham, AL 35233
(205) 934-9999
Best in: Rheumatology

UNIVERSITY OF TEXAS
(M. D. Anderson Cancer
Center)
1515 Holcombe Boulevard
Houston, TX 77030
(713) 792-2121
Best in: Cancer, gynecology,
otolaryngology, urology

WEST

CHILDREN'S HOSPITAL LOS
ANGELES
4650 Sunset Boulevard
Los Angeles, CA 90027
(213) 660-2450
Best in: Pediatrics

CRAIG HOSPITAL
3425 South Clarkson Street
Englewood, CO 80110
(303) 789-8000
Best in: Rehabilitation

RANCHO LOS AMIGOS
MEDICAL CENTER
7601 E. Imperial Highway
Downey, CA 90242
(310) 940-7041
Best in: Rehabilitation

SAN FRANCISCO GENERAL
HOSPITAL

1001 Potrero Avenue
San Francisco, CA 94110
(415) 206-8000
Best in: AIDS

STANFORD UNIVERSITY
HOSPITAL
300 Pasteur Drive
Stanford, CA 94305
(415) 723-1245
Best in: Cancer, cardiology,
urology

UCLA MEDICAL CENTER
(JULES STEIN EYE
INSTITUTE)
10833 LeConte Avenue
Los Angeles, CA 90024
(310) 825-9111
Best in: AIDS, gastroenterology,
geriatrics, neurology,
ophthalmology, otolaryngology,
psychiatry, rheumatology,
urology

UNIVERSITY OF
CALIFORNIA
SAN FRANCISCO MEDICAL
CENTER
505 Parnassus Avenue
San Francisco, CA 94143
(415) 476-1000
Best in: AIDS, endocrinology,
neurology

UNIVERSITY OF
WASHINGTON MEDICAL
CENTER
1959 N.E. Pacific Street
Seattle, WA 98195
(206) 548-3300
Best in: Rehabilitation, urology

# *Appendix E*

## SOURCES OF MEDICAL SURVEYS

*Taking Charge
of Your Medical Fate*
Lawrence Horowitz, M.D.
Random House, 1986
New York, NY

*The Best in Medicine*
Herbert J. Dietrich, M.D.
Harmony Publishing, 1986
New York, NY

"The Best in Medicine"
John Pekkanen
*Town and Country*, 1984
New York, NY

"The Twenty-Five
Best Hospitals"

*U.S. News & World Report,*
June 1992
2400 N Street, NW
Washington, DC

"The 44 Best Hospitals
in America"
M. Abrams
A Special G.M. Report
*Family Circle*, 1983
110 Fifth Avenue
New York, NY

*Health Care U.S.A.*
Jean Carper
Prentice-Hall, 1987
New York, NY

# Appendix F

## PHARMACEUTICAL REFERENCES

*About Your Medicines*
U.S. Pharmacopeia Dispensing
Information
Mack Printing Company
Easton, PA 18042

*Compendium of Drug Therapy*
Biomedical Information
Corporation
800 Second Ave.
New York, NY 10017

*Complete Guide to Prescription
& Non-Prescription Drugs*
by H. Winter Griffith
The Body Press/Perigee
Putnam Publishing Co.
200 Madison Ave.
New York, NY 10016

*Consumer Reports Books:
Drug Information for the
Consumer*
Mount Vernon, NY 10551

*1991 Drugs Available Abroad*
& Gale Research, Inc.
835 Penodscote Blvd.
Detroit, MI 48226

*Drug Interaction Facts:
Facts and Comparisons*
J. B. Lippincott Co.

111 W. Port Plaza, Suite 423
St. Louis, MO 63146

*The Food & Drug Interaction
Guide*
By Brian Morgan, 1986
Simon & Schuster
1230 Avenue of the Americas
New York, NY 10020

*A Guide to
Antimicrobial Therapy*
Antimicrobial Therapy
PO Box 34456
West Bethesda, MD 20817-
0456

*Modell's Drugs in Current Use*
Springer Publishing Co., 1992
New York, NY 10012

*Mosby's 1992 Nursing Drug
Reference*
Roth, Linda, Mosby Publishing
St. Louis, MO 63146

*The New Consumer Drug Digest*
American Society of Hospital
Pharmacists, 1985
Bethesda, MD 20814

*Pharmacopeia*
Mack Publishing Company

46 Park Ave.
New York, NY 10016

*Physician's Desk Reference (PDR)*
Medical Economics, Inc.
Oredell, NJ 07649

*USP Drug Information Division*
1206 Twinbrook Parkway
Rockville, MD 20852

# *Appendix G*

## PHYSICIAN SPECIALTIES

| Specialist | Specialization Area |
|---|---|
| Acupuncturist | Pain Control |
| Allergist | Allergic diseases, allergies |
| Anesthesiologist | Anesthesia, respiratory system |
| Cardiologist | Heart and vascular system |
| Dermatologist | Skin disease and disorders |
| Endocrinologist | Glands, hormones, and metabolism |
| Gastroenterologist | Intestinal tract |
| Geriatrics | Treatment of aged |
| Gynecologist | Female reproductive system |
| Hematologist | Blood and blood-forming organ disorders |
| Immunologist | Autoimmune diseases |
| Infectious disease | Infectious and contagious diseases |
| Internist | Internal disorders |
| Laryngologist | Throat disorders |
| Nephrologist | Kidney disorders |
| Neurologist | Nervous system diseases |
| Neurosurgeon | Surgery in the brain and spine |
| Nuclear medicine | Radioactive medicine |
| Obstetrician | Pregnancy and childbirth |
| Oncologist | Cancer and tumors |
| Ophthalmologist | Eye diseases |
| Orthopedist | Bones, muscles, joints, and spine disorders |
| Osteopath | Musculoskeletal system |
| Otologist | Ear disorders |
| Otorhinolaryngologist | Ears, nose, throat (ENT) |
| Pathologist | Laboratory testing and autopsies |
| Pediatrician | Babies and children |
| Plastic surgeon | Reconstruction of body deformities |
| Podiatrist | Foot and ankle disorders |

| | |
|---|---|
| Proctologist | Colon and rectal disease |
| Psychiatrist | Emotional and behavioral disorders |
| Physiatrist | Rehabilitation and therapy |
| Pulmonary | Lung disorders |
| Radiologist | Diagnostic and therapeutic radiology |
| Rheumatologist | Rheumatoid arthritis, inflammation |
| Rhinologist | Treatment of nose |
| Thoracic surgeon | Surgery in chest area |
| Thoracic-cardiac surgeon | Surgery of heart, chest, and lung |
| Urologist | Urinary tract and prostate disease |

# Appendix H

## A PATIENT'S BILL OF RIGHTS*

1. The patient has the right to considerate and respectful care.

2. The patient has the right to and is encouraged to obtain from physicians and other direct caregivers relevant, current, and understandable information concerning diagnosis, treatment, and prognosis.

   Except in emergencies when the patient lacks decision-making capacity and the need for treatment is urgent, the patient is entitled to the opportunity to discuss and request information related to the specific procedures and/or treatments, the risks involved, the possible length of recuperation, and the medically reasonable alternatives and their accompanying risks and benefits.

   Patients have the right to know the identity of physicians, nurses, and others involved in their care, as well as when those involved are students, residents, or other trainees. The patient also has the right to know the immediate and long-term financial implications of treatment choices, insofar as they are known.

3. The patient has the right to make decisions about the plan of care prior to and during the course of treatment and to refuse a recommended treatment or plan of care to the extent permitted by law and hospital policy and to be informed of the medical consequences of this action. In case of such refusal, the patient is

---

*These rights can be exercised on the patient's behalf by a designated surrogate or proxy decision maker if the patient lacks decision-making capacity, is legally incompetent, or is a minor.

entitled to other appropriate care and services that the hospital provides or transfer to another hospital. The hospital should notify patients of any policy that might affect patient choice within the institution.

4. The patient has the right to have an advance directive (such as a living will, health care proxy, or durable power of attorney for health care) concerning treatment or designating a surrogate decision maker with the expectation that the hospital will honor the intent of that directive to the extent permitted by law and hospital policy.

   Health care institutions must advise patients of their rights under state law and hospital policy to make informed medical choices, ask if the patient has an advance directive, and include that information in patient records. The patient has the right to timely information about hospital policy that may limit its ability to implement fully a legally valid advance directive.

5. The patient has the right to every consideration of privacy. Case discussion, consultation, examination, and treatment should be conducted so as to protect each patient's privacy.

6. The patient has the right to expect that all communications and records pertaining to his/her care will be treated as confidential by the hospital, except in cases such as suspected abuse and public health hazards when reporting is permitted or required by law. The patient has the right to expect that the hospital will emphasize the confidentiality of this information when it releases it to any other parties entitled to review information in these records.

7. The patient has the right to review the records pertaining to his/her medical care and to have the information explained or interpreted as necessary, except when restricted by law.

8. The patient has the right to expect that, within its capacity and policies, a hospital will make reasonable response to the request of a patient for appropriate and medically indicated care and services. The hospital must provide evaluation, service, and/or referral as indicated by the urgency of the case. When medically appropriate and legally permissible, or when a patient has so requested, a patient may be transferred to another facility. The institution to which the patient is to be transferred must first have accepted the patient for transfer. The patient must also have the benefit of complete information and

explanation concerning the need for, risks, benefits, and alternatives to such a transfer.

9. The patient has the right to ask and be informed of the existence of business relationships among the hospital, educational institutions, other health care providers, or payers that may influence the patient's treatment and care.

10. The patient has the right to consent to or decline to participate in proposed research studies or human experimentation affecting care and treatment or requiring direct patient involvement, and to have those studies fully explained prior to consent. A patient who declines to participate in research or experimentation is entitled to the most effective care that the hospital can otherwise provide.

11. The patient has the right to expect reasonable continuity of care when appropriate and to be informed by physicians and other caregivers of available and realistic patient care options when hospital care is no longer appropriate.

12. The patient has the right to be informed of hospital policies and practices that relate to patient care, treatment, and responsibilities. The patient has the right to be informed of available resources for resolving disputes, grievances, and conflicts, such as ethics committees, patient representatives, or other mechanisms available in the institution. The patient has the right to be informed of the hospital's charges for services and available payment methods.

---

*A Patient's Bill of Rights* was first adopted by the American Hospital Association in 1973. This revision was approved by the AHA Board of Trustees on October 21, 1992.

# References

Abrams, Maxine, "The 44 Best Hospitals in America." *Family Circle*, May 1983, 141.

Carson, Ben, *Think Big: Unleashing Your Potential for Excellence*, Grand Rapids, Michigan: Zondervan Publishing House, 1992.

Carter, Jean. *Health Care U.S.A.* New York: Prentice-Hall Press, 1987.

DeVita, Vincent. "New System Offers Laetrile Cancer Data." *Chicago Tribune*, February 2, 1985, Section 6, 2.

Dietrich, Herbert. *The Best in Medicine*. New York: Harmony Books, 1986.

Farnum, Angel. "Why Didn't My Doctors Listen to Me?" *Good Housekeeping*, April 1992, 103.

Hales, Dianna. "The Disease That Fuels the Doctors." *Good Housekeeping*, April 1992, 62−64.

Horowitz, Lawrence. *Taking Charge of Your Medical Fate*. New York: Random House, 1986.

Johnson, Paul. *Conquering Cancer*. Grand Rapids, Michigan: Zondervan Publishing House, 1992.

Kushner, Harold. *When Bad Things Happen to Good People*. New York: Avon Books, 1981.

Levin, Arthur. *Talk Back to Your Doctor*. New York: Doubleday and Company, 9, 1977.

Levitt, Paul. *You Can Make It Back: Coping With Serious Illness*. New York: R. R. Donnelly & Sons Co., 1985.

Pekkanen, John. "The Best Medical Specialists in the U.S." *Town and Country*, 165, June 1984.

Robert Wood Johnson Foundation. *Challenges in Health Care: A Chart Book Perspective*. Princeton, New Jersey: 1991.

"The Twenty-Five Best Hospitals." *U.S. News & World Report*, August 1991.

Yancy, Philip. *Where Is God When It Hurts*. Grand Rapids, Michigan: Zondervan Publishing House, 1990.

# Endnotes

[1]Horowitz, Lawrence. *Taking Charge of Your Medical Fate*. New York: Random House, 1986.

[2]Levin, Arthur. *Talk Back to Your Doctor*. New York: Doubleday and Company, 1977, p. 9.

[3]"Kids at Risk—The Shame of Emergency Medicine." *U.S. News & World Report*. January 27, 1992 (reprint), p. 1.

[4]"Artificial Joints Help Arthritis Sufferers Regain Independence." *The LaPorte Herald-Argus*. LaPorte, Indiana, October 7, 1991.

[5]"The Case for Health Care Technology" (brochure). HIMA (Health Industry Manufacturers Association), Washington, D.C., p. 2.

[6]Hales, Diana. "The Disease That Fuels the Doctors." *Good Housekeeping*, April 1992, pp. 62–64.

[7]"Quackery in Cancer Nutrition Harms 50,000 Persons a Year." *The Daily Sentinel-Tribune*. Bowling Green, Ohio, February 7, 1985.

[8]DeVita, Vincent. "New System Offers Laetrile Cancer Data." *Chicago Tribune*, Section 6, February 2, 1985, p. 2.

[9]Pekkanen, John. "The Best Medical Specialists in the U.S." *Town and Country*, June 1984, p. 165.

[10]Dietrich, Herbert. *The Best in Medicine*. New York: Harmony Books, 1986, p. x.

[11]Carson, Ben. *Think Big: Unleashing Your Potential for Excellence*. Grand Rapids, Michigan: Zondervan Publishing House, 1992, pp. 242–243.

[12]Moran, Claudia. "HMO's Try to Measure and Regard 'Doctor Quality.'" *Medical Economics*. April 6, 1992, p. 207.

[13]Egerton, M.D., John R. "The Key to Lower Health Costs: A Doctor's Educated Guess." *Medical Economics*. February 17, 1991, p. 199.

[14]*People's Medical Society Newsletter*, M561, p. 5.

[15]Ibid.

[16]Health Care Financing Administration. *Medicare Hospital Mortality Information, 1986*. Department of Health & Human Services, Washington, D.C. 20201, p. 1.

[17]The Public Citizen Health Research Group. *Health Letter*. May 1990, Vol. 6, No. 5, p. 1.

[18]"America's Best Hospitals." *U. S. News & World Report.* June 15, 1992 (reprint), p. 3.

[19]Dietrich, Herbert J., M.D., and Virginia H. Biddle. *The Best in Medicine.* New York: Harmony Books, 1986, p. 6.

[20]Cohan, Carol: Primm, June; and James Jude. *A Patient's Guide to Heart Surgery.* New York: Harper Perennial, Division of HarperCollins, 1991, pp. 41, 43.

For information on speaking engagements or seminars (conflict, stress, health, motivation, team building, leadership, communications, self-management, problem solving and decision making, and so forth) for your company or organization, write:

Dr. Dan Tomal
P.O. Box 725
LaPorte, IN 46350